Wound Management in the Horse

Editor

EARL M. GAUGHAN

VETERINARY CLINICS OF NORTH AMERICA: EQUINE PRACTICE

www.vetequine.theclinics.com

Consulting Editor
THOMAS J. DIVERS

December 2018 • Volume 34 • Number 3

ELSEVIER

1600 John F. Kennedy Boulevard • Suite 1800 • Philadelphia, Pennsylvania, 19103-2899

http://www.vetequine.theclinics.com

VETERINARY CLINICS OF NORTH AMERICA: EQUINE PRACTICE Volume 34, Number 3
December 2018 ISSN 0749-0739, ISBN-13: 978-0-323-64324-5

Editor: Colleen Dietzler
Developmental Editor: Donald Mumford

Veterinary Clinics of North America: Equine Practice (ISSN 0749-0739) is published in April, August, and December by Elsevier Inc., 360 Park Avenue South, New York, NY 10010-1710. Business and Editorial Offices: 1600 John F. Kennedy Blvd., Suite 1800, Philadelphia, PA 19103-2899. Subscription prices are $281.00 per year (domestic individuals), $536.00 per year (domestic institutions), $100.00 per year (domestic students/residents), $328.00 per year (Canadian individuals), $675.00 per year (Canadian institutions), $365.00 per year (international individuals), $675.00 per year (international institutions), and $180.00 per year (international and Canadian students/residents). To receive student/resident rate, orders must be accompanied by name of affiliated institution, date of term, and the signature of program/residency coordinator on institution letterhead. Orders will be billed at individual rate until proof of status is received. Foreign air speed delivery is included in all Clinics subscription prices. All prices are subject to change without notice. **POSTMASTER:** Send address changes to Veterinary Clinics of North America: Equine Practice, 3251 Riverport Lane, Maryland Heights, MO 63043. Customer Service (orders, claims, online, change of address): Elsevier Health Sciences Division, Subscription Customer **Service, 3251 Riverport Lane, Maryland Heights, MO 63043. Tel: 1-800-654-2452 (U.S. and Canada); 314-447-8871 (outside U.S. and Canada). Fax: 314-447-8029. E-mail: journalscustomerservice-usa@elsevier.com (for print support);** E-mail: **journalsonlinesupport-usa@elsevier.com (for online support).**

Reprints. For copies of 100 or more of articles in this publication, please contact the Commercial Reprints Department, Elsevier Inc., 360 Park Avenue South, New York, NY 10010-1710. Tel.: 212-633-3874; Fax: 212-633-3820; E-mail: reprints@elsevier.com.

Veterinary Clinics of North America: Equine Practice is covered in MEDLINE/PubMed (Index Medicus), Excerpta Medica, Current Contents/Agriculture, Biology and Environmental Sciences, and ISI.

Contributors

CONSULTING EDITOR

THOMAS J. DIVERS, DVM
Diplomate, American College of Veterinary Internal Medicine; Diplomate, American College of Veterinary Emergency and Critical Care; Steffen Professor of Veterinary Medicine, Section of Large Animal Medicine, College of Veterinary Medicine, Cornell University, Ithaca, New York, USA

EDITOR

EARL M. GAUGHAN, DVM
Diplomate, American College of Veterinary Surgeons; Equine Professional Services Veterinarian, Merck Animal Health, Madison, New Jersey, USA

AUTHORS

LINDA A. DAHLGREN, DVM, PhD
Diplomate, American College of Veterinary Surgeons; Associate Professor, Department of Large Animal Clinical Sciences, Virginia-Maryland College of Veterinary Medicine, Virginia Tech, Blacksburg, Virginia, USA

RANDY B. EGGLESTON, DVM
Diplomate, American College of Veterinary Surgeons; Clinical Professor, Department of Large Animal Medicine, College of Veterinary Medicine, University of Georgia, Athens, Georgia, USA

KARL E. FREES, DVM, MS
Diplomate, American College of Veterinary Surgeons; Wilhite & Frees Equine Hospital, Peculiar, Missouri, USA

EARL M. GAUGHAN, DVM
Diplomate, American College of Veterinary Surgeons; Equine Professional Services Veterinarian, Merck Animal Health, Madison, New Jersey, USA

R. REID HANSON, DVM
Diplomate, American College of Veterinary Surgeons; Diplomate, American College of Veterinary Emergency and Critical Care; Professor of Equine Surgery, Department of Clinical Sciences, J.T. Vaughan Teaching Hospital, Auburn University College of Veterinary Medicine, Auburn, Alabama, USA

LOUIS KAMUS, DMV, MSc
Resident in Equine Surgery, Clinical Sciences, Faculté de médecine vétérinaire, Université de Montréal, Saint-Hyacinthe, Quebec, Canada

LEANN KUEBELBECK, DVM
Diplomate, American College of Veterinary Surgeons; President, Co-Owner, Brandon Equine Medical Center, Brandon, Florida, USA

BRITTA S. LEISE, DVM, PhD
Diplomate, American College of Veterinary Surgeons-Large Animal; Assistant Professor, Equine Surgery, Veterinary Clinical Sciences, School of Veterinary Medicine, Louisiana State University, Baton Rouge, Louisiana, USA

ELSA K. LUDWIG, DVM, MS
Associate, Vermont Large Animal Clinic, Equine Hospital, Milton, Vermont, USA

MICHAEL MAHER, DVM
Diplomate, American College of Veterinary Surgeons-Large Animal; Staff Surgeon, Co-Owner, Brandon Equine Medical Center, Brandon, Florida, USA

CHRISTINE THEORET, DMV, PhD
Diplomate, American College of Veterinary Surgeons; Professor and Dean, Faculté de médecine vétérinaire, Université de Montréal, Saint-Hyacinthe, Quebec Canada

PHILIP D. VAN HARREVELD, DVM, MS
Diplomate, American College of Veterinary Surgeons; Owner, Vermont Large Animal Clinic, Equine Hospital, Milton, Vermont, USA

Contents

An accurate and timely diagnosis of the systemic and local tissue influences of a wound are essential to target successful treatment measures
and reach the best result for an affected horse. A complete physical examination should be completed for any wounded horse and appropriate systemic therapies instituted. Visual and manipulative examinations aid in the
complete understanding of wounded tissues. Imaging and invasive diagnostic techniques also have value in determining the extent of a wound.
Considering what tissues are involved from an inside–out perspective
can assist in developing a complete diagnosis.

The goal of wound cleansing and care is the control or removal of tissue
infection to allow healing in the most functional, cosmetic, fastest, and least
expensive manner possible. This is accomplished through the removal of
debris and necrotic tissue while reducing the bacterial load via careful
use of mechanical techniques and cleaning agents, accepting that
some level of tissue trauma will result. Keep in mind that the benefit of a clean
wound must be weighed against the trauma inflicted in the process of
cleansing. Veterinary health care professionals should take hygienic steps
to reduce hospital-acquired infections and zoonotic disease transmission.

Topical therapies are used in equine wound healing to clean and decontaminate the wound environment after acute injury, to promote healing,
and to decrease the risk of infection once the wound has initially been
treated. Evolving antibiotic resistance has prompted judicious use of systemic antimicrobials, particularly in the treatment of local infections, such
as wounds. The use of topical antiseptics to disinfect acute wounds and
topical antimicrobials to manage chronic wounds is necessary to achieve
successful healing. In addition, many topical medications can alter the
wound environment to promote rapid and effective wound healing.

This article aims to help the practitioner by providing the tools to decide
which type of closure or healing is best in a given situation. An overview
of the main criteria and the different approaches to wound closure is presented. Each wound must be considered as a unique problem that

Wound Management: Wounds with Special Challenges   511

Randy B. Eggleston

Distal limb wounds in horses heal substantially different than trunk wounds, commonly resulting in exuberant granulation tissue and exposed and sequestered bone. Surgical intervention of severe rectovaginal lacerations in the mare should be delayed until the tissues have heeled and scar tissue has remodeled. Wounds resulting in severe hemorrhage require appropriate emergent fluid therapy and potentially transfusion therapy.

Nonhealing Wounds of the Equine Limb   539

Michael Maher and Leann Kuebelbeck

Nonhealing wounds present a common challenge to the equine practitioner. An underlying source of inflammation and infection is almost always present and needs to be resolved for healing to proceed. Wound débridement is the mainstay for this resolution. In addition, wound closure, wound dressings, and skin grafts can be used to achieve successful wound healing.

Equine Wound Management: Bandages, Casts, and External Support   557

Randy B. Eggleston

Successful management of equine wounds relies on knowledge of the stages of wound healing, factors that can alter those stages, how healing stages can be manipulated, and adherence to the principles of wound healing. Challenges that complicate wound management include the inability to immobilize and/or confine equine patients, and maintain a clean environment during the critical initial stages of healing. Because of these challenges, the equine practitioner relies heavily on bandaging and external coaptation techniques to successfully treat and manage wounds. The type of bandage used is dictated by the region of the body that is injured.

Equine Wounds over Synovial Structures   575

Elsa K. Ludwig and Philip D. van Harreveld

Equine septic synovitis commonly occurs secondary to traumatic wounds. The distal limbs of horses have minimal soft tissue protection, thus wounds in these areas are more likely to involve adjacent synovial structures. Synovial sepsis can be debilitating due to difficulties clearing established infections and the degenerative changes that result from ongoing inflammation. Prompt diagnosis allows for immediate treatment, improving the prognosis. Goals for successful treatment of infected synovial structures due to wounds include early and accurate recognition of the condition, rapid resolution of pain and inflammation, complete elimination of microorganisms, appropriate wound healing, and a timely return to function.

Suitable use of prophylactic antimicrobial drugs for wounds depends on the accurate selection of appropriate antibiotics, dosing regimen, and duration of use. Regional intravenous delivery and intraosseous infusion of antibiotics are pivotal to a successful outcome for deep-rooted infections, inadequately perfused tissue, and infected wounds containing biofilm. Antibiotic-impregnated polymethylmethacrylate beads are predominantly helpful for wounds that have a poor blood supply and for those containing surgical implants that must remain in place.

Wound management in horses can strike fear in some and passion in others. Wounds are common injuries in horses of all descriptions and requires exceptional knowledge and care to achieve a successful outcome. New treatments to overcome the critical challenges with equine wounds are always desired: managing dehisced and/or nonhealing wounds, managing exuberant granulation tissue, and ultimately achieving a functional tissue coverage. Regenerative medicine represents a broad set of tools with great promise to manipulate the deficiencies recognized in equine wound healing and improve the outcome.

VETERINARY CLINICS OF
NORTH AMERICA: EQUINE PRACTICE

RELATED SERIES

Veterinary Clinics of North America: Food Animal Practice

THE CLINICS ARE NOW AVAILABLE ONLINE!
Access your subscription at:
www.theclinics.com

Preface

Wound Management

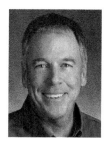

Earl M. Gaughan, DVM
Editor

Wounds, of many origins and conformations, are common for horses and show no bias by age, breed, sex, or athletic pursuit. Veterinarians develop preferences in diagnostic and treatment methods through education, experience, and discussion. So much of wound management evolves from the basic tenets of "First, do no harm." With this in mind, the authors of this issue of *Veterinary Clinics of North America: Equine Practice* have used known medical science combined with their wealth of hands-on experience to offer practical, usable information for the diagnosis and management of equine wounds.

The authors have described and encouraged early, accurate diagnoses. Gentle and thorough cleansing, with close tissue observation and detection of potential wound and contamination complications, are keys to sound early wound management. Aggressive detection of deep and vital tissue injury/penetration will allow initiation of targeted, aggressive therapies, which is ultimately the key to successful management and return to intended use. Some wounds present specific challenges that may not be common. Suggestions are offered for decisions about closing wounds, managing synovial and bone involvement, and when limb motion can lead to potential nonhealing concerns. Agents that can safely, and efficaciously, be topically placed on wounds are always important considerations, and appropriate selections are vital when managing an equine wound. Considerations of systemic support for a wounded horse are also offered here as well as the new "frontier" of regenerative medical applications to wounded tissues.

Managing equine wounds can be very frustrating for the horse, the owner, and the veterinarian. No formula for action is going to work for every horse or for every similar wound. Keeping the basic tenets of wound management in mind and working with experienced advice from colleagues can help reach the best outcomes in the most expedient amount of time. The authors throughout this issue have put great effort into presenting information, and offering their preferences, with regard to likely

Vet Clin Equine 34 (2018) ix–x
https://doi.org/10.1016/j.cveq.2018.09.001
0749-0739/18/© 2018 Published by Elsevier Inc.

success in returning wounded horses to their intended roles and also with attention to what is sound and cost-effective medical science.

I would like to thank Dr Tom Divers for the invitation to help with this issue. He has been there from the beginnings of my career to today, as a mentor, a guide, and a friend. My thanks also go to the Editors of *Veterinary Clinics of North America: Equine Practice* for their help, patience, and encouragement. I am always and forever thankful for Kathy, my rock, and Michael and Jesse, my constant sources of inspiration.

Earl M. Gaughan, DVM
Equine Professional Services Veterinarian
Merck Animal Health
2 Giralda Farms
Madison, NJ 07940, USA

E-mail address:
earl.gaughan@merck.com

Diagnostic Approaches to Understanding Equine Limb Wounds

Earl M. Gaughan, DVM*

KEYWORDS

- Early diagnosis • Visual examination • Manipulative examination
- Essential to understand all injured tissue

KEY POINTS

- Early diagnosis and treatment lead to best outcomes after wounding.
- Careful attention to all tissues involved in a wound can lead to best management decisions.
- Interpreting a wound from the deepest affected tissues out to the skin surface is important for a complete diagnosis.
- A complete physical examination is indicated for every wounded horse.
- Visual, palpation, and manipulative examinations help to determine the complete wound diagnosis.

Horses are prone to wounding and serious secondary repercussions, often owing to their innate inquisitiveness followed by rapid and aggressive flight from fright protective impulses. Unfortunately, horses' limbs do not have substantial protection with muscle or other tissue, which can often satisfactorily be repaired; and therefore, distal limb tissues under the skin are exposed to potential serious and long-lasting complications from wounding. The "1 wound–1 scar" concept described by Peacock[1] years ago still applies today, and especially so for horses. Tissues from the skin to the depths of a wound tend to heal as one, through the progressive stages of wound healing. Equine limbs, with a great capability of generating granulation tissue, can often have long-term function inhibited by this tendency to have 1 scar. This concern is long term for wounds on the flexor surface of the distal limb where scar tissue and

Disclosure Statement: The author has no relationship with a commercial company that has a direct financial interest in subject matter or materials discussed in article or with a company making a competing product.

Equine Veterinary Professional Services, Merck Animal Health, Merck Animal Health, 2 Giralda Farms, Madison, NJ 07940, USA

* 5860 Sioux Drive, Sedalia, CO 80135.

E-mail address: earl.gaughan@merck.com

fibrous adhesions can disrupt normal mechanical function of flexor tendons and the various ligamentous structures. As Dr Marvin Beeman has long described (Beeman MG. Personal communication, 2006), normal form is required for normal function. Thus, management of wounds of the equine distal limb often becomes a race against time and the tendencies toward 1 scar. Preserving normal limb function is a matter of preserving and returning wounded tissues to as close to normal form as possible.

Timely and accurate assessment of an equine limb wound is essential to achieve a satisfactory outcome for the horse and the owner. Delays and misinterpretations can result in the loss of normal tissue and normal limb function, as well as secondary complications like sepsis and fibrosis, which can broaden the influence of a local wound on total limb function. Avoiding long-term repercussions after an acute injury can often be achieved with an early understanding of what tissues are injured and to what extent the involved tissues are disrupted. The location of a wound and magnitude of skin and likely deeper tissue involvement, as well as what, if any, tissue has been lost are important early things to note. Consideration of likely complications from motion at a wound's anatomic location at the time of examination and through the needed time to achieve healing will also dictate management techniques (see Randy B. Eggleston's article, "Equine Wound Management: Bandages, Casts, and External Support," in this issue).

HISTORY

An accurate history can be a solid asset when evaluating a limb wound. Often an owner account of an injury incident does not fit well with the wound a veterinarian may be looking at in real time. This discrepancy is not usually an intent to mislead by the horse owner, but can simply be a lack of observation or a misunderstanding of what happened and when. Wounds that are acutely noticed may not necessarily have occurred in the recent past. A visual examination, followed by a thorough physical examination often can make this determination, but all accurate information regarding how a wound occurred, and when, is important to overall medical management (**Boxes 1–3**).

Noting the signalment of a wounded horse may not reveal anything specific to the nature and severity of a wound. However, age and potential age-related metabolic disorders may influence the management and progression of wound healing, and therefore a horse's age is worth understanding on initial examination.

Some historical action can be disruptive to a timely and accurate, complete wound diagnosis. Owners frequently feel compelled to do something, and often that something involves the topical application of a wound dressing in the form of ointments, powders, or solutions. Many of these available compounds are of various colors and most are of dubious indications. When possible, it seems to be wise to council an owner of a wounded horse to delay application of any topical substances until a

---

Box 1
Visual signs of an acute wound (day 1)
Active hemorrhage
Presence of "fresh" debris
Laceration: sharp tissue margins
Abrasion/tearing wound: tissues may have defined, yet frayed margins
Acute pain from wounding

Box 2
Visual signs at days 2 to 3 after wounding

Serum or other fluid (ie, synovial fluid) presence replaces frank blood

Early exudate (purulent) is possible

Swelling

Lameness (indicates further examination of structural tissues)

---

veterinarian can complete a thorough physical and wound examination. It is very frustrating to try to remove a substance that may occlude visual examination, stain tissues, and potentially harm deep, wounded vital tissues. Likely nothing is superior to good hygiene practices with sterile solutions or clean water, especially as a prelude to veterinary examination (see Karl E. Frees' article, "Equine Practice on Wound Management: Wound Cleansing and Hygiene," in this issue). It is often good advice to a horse owner to cover a limb wound with a sterile, or even clean, bandage, as a triage maneuver to address the time between a phone call and when a veterinarian can evaluate the horse and the wound. This step can reduce the likelihood of further trauma and contamination before appropriate wound examination and care can take place.

COMPLETE PHYSICAL EXAMINATION AND PATIENT RESTRAINT

Examination of a wound should begin with an overall examination of the wounded horse. A thorough physical examination is indicated. Assessment of the horse is often accomplished quickly and appropriately for the situation at hand and should include systemic evaluation such that threats to overall health are not missed owing to specific attention to the wound itself. Assessment of vital signs and other systemic factors can lead to a more thorough understanding of a horse's current health status. Tachycardia, fever, mentation changes, and other systemic indicators may dictate the necessity of further investigation of wound influence beyond just local tissue disruption.

Noting the severity of lameness after wounding is usually intuitive on first visual observation of an affected horse. Horses with grades 4 to 5, out of 5, on the American Association of Equine Practitioners lameness scale should not be moved from where they are found until a complete veterinary examination has been completed. Horses with less severe lameness can be confounding at times, because acute wounding that involves synovial or other vital support tissues may not demonstrate lameness that is consistent with deeper tissue injury. Similarly, more chronic wounds into these tissues that establish drainage through the wound, will not be as lame as a horse with a closed septic compartment (see Elsa K. Ludwig and Philip D. van Harreveld's article, "Equine Wounds over Synovial Structures," in this issue). When evaluating lameness secondary to wounding, all possibilities must be evaluated and the most severe repercussions considered possible until proven otherwise.

Box 3
Clinical signs of day 3 or more after wounding

Granulation tissue may become evident (fibroblasts arrive in wound site on days 3–5)

Wound margin contraction may be present

Deep-seated sepsis may be present (ie, pain and lameness)

Appropriate restraint is needed to accomplish accurate diagnostic interpretations. Restraint can be as simple as having a competent handler on a lead line and halter, but frequently chemical restraint means are necessary. Individual veterinarians have personally preferred methods and drugs, and several factors are common when selecting what will be used for chemical restraint. Duration of time needed to complete the diagnostic and treatment tasks should be estimated when making drug choices. It is also important to avoid making the situation more complicated. Avoiding excessive ataxia from sedation is important for the horse, the handler, and the veterinarian. Careful sedative/tranquilizing drug use is essential. Most commonly, agents like xylazine and detomidine should be administered in doses below those described for preanesthesia on the labels. Xylazine (0.2–1.1 mg/kg administered intravenously [IV] or intramuscularly)[2] will typically restrain an adult horse in place but also produce some degree of mental stupor and ataxia. The same can be described for detomidine (0.005–0.02 mg/kg administered IV or intramuscularly).[2] Similar considerations should be made for the use of analgesic agents like butorphanol (0.05–0.1 mg/kg administered IV).[2] Also, it should be understood that butorphanol will potentiate the sedative and ataxia-inducing effects of xylazine and detomidine when administered in combination. Systemic influences of these sedative agents on vital signs (ie, reducing heart rate) should be kept in mind as data from a total examination are summarized and interpreted. Tranquilizing medications, like acepromazine, should be used with care and understanding of expected results, because restraint can be difficult to obtain when these drugs are administered to a wounded horse already agitated, and/or if negative cardiovascular effects of wounding are a concern.

Systemic administration of nonsteroidal antiinflammatory drugs does not often complicate wound examination; however, a complete physical examination will determine safety of using these drugs. Influences of nonsteroidal antiinflammatory drugs on wound healing are discussed in R. Reid Hanson's article, "Medical Therapy in Equine Wound Management," in this issue.

Regional and local anesthesia of wounded limbs should be performed with caution if any supportive tissues (ie, bone, ligament, tendon) are considered to be involved in the wound. Complete local anesthesia can remove the innate protective mechanisms of an injured horse, and potential decompensation of a wounded limb should be evaluated and avoided.

FIRST AID

Rendering first aid can postpone complete wound examination. Controlling voluminous hemorrhage, providing structural support, neurologic assessment, and life-saving systemic treatment should be prioritized over a complete understanding of wounded tissues. A complete physical examination and the initial wound examination can help to determine these appropriate delays in wound management. The realities of the situation may alter what would be ideal for wound examination and treatment scenarios. Timing to an accurate wound diagnosis can be critical to long-term success and return to function, but delays in this assessment may be necessary at times when systemic factors so dictate.

DIAGNOSTIC EXERCISES

As a guideline, it makes sense to consider a wound as having occurred "from the outside "in"" (ie, from the skin surface to the depth of the wound), and complete diagnostic understanding of a wound should be "from the inside out." In other words, a complete understanding of a wound should concentrate on knowing the deepest reach of tissue disruption and each individual tissue between there and the skin surface (**Fig. 1**). This can be accomplished in a number of manners, from the simplest visual observations to the most intricate of manipulative and imaging modalities.

It is essential to have the most thorough understanding possible of the status of any vital tissues associated with a wound. Vital tissues in this regard are vascular, neurologic, and structural (bone, ligament, tendon, and synovial; see Elsa K. Ludwig and Philip D. van Harreveld's article, "Equine Wounds over Synovial Structures," and Randy B. Eggleston's article, "Wound Management: Wounds with Special Challenges," in this issue). Vascular tissue is most commonly a consideration when hemorrhage is notable, if not excessive. In this circumstance, first aid initiatives directed at hemorrhage control and systemic cardiovascular support are appropriate (ie, pressure bandaging; IV fluid therapy; see Randy B. Eggleston's article, "Equine Wound Management: Bandages, Casts, and External Support," in this issue). In the less common situation where circumferential wounding may affect limb vasculature and potential perfusion of the limb distal to a wound, it is important to recognize that a complete understanding of subsequent and future blood flow to the affected aspects of the limb may be delayed for up to 5 to 7 days. Therefore, in this circumstance delayed wound management may be prudent (see **Boxes 1–3**; see Louis

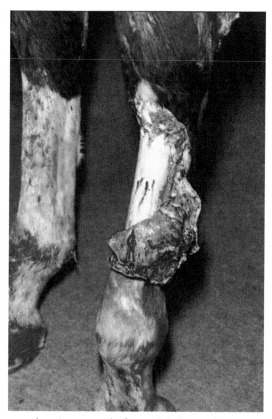

Fig. 1. Severe metatarsal region wound of an adult horse: determining what tissues are wounded is essential for appropriate management decisions. Consider tissues from the outside in. Tissues involved in this wound include skin, subcutaneous tissues, extensor tendon, periosteum, and superficial cortical bone. Potential "vital" tissue involvement includes the tarsometatarsal joint, metatarsophalangeal joint, and digital flexor tendon sheath.

Kamus and Christine Theoret's article, "Choosing the Best Approach to Wound Management and Closure," in this issue).

VISUAL EXAMINATION

Not all wounded tissues can be visualized in every equine limb wound. However, a good initial examination should evaluate wounded tissues as completely as possible without doing further harm to vital structures (see **Fig. 1**). Taking a close initial look and continuing the visual examination throughout the cleansing process (see Karl E. Frees' article, "Equine Practice on Wound Management: Wound Cleansing and Hygiene," in this issue) should not be ignored as a valuable tool. Useful information can be missed simply by not carefully looking at a wound. Once again, careful restraint is needed to closely visualize limb wounds.

The initial examination should also include consideration of the factors that have the potential to delay or interfere with wound healing. Contamination with foreign materials and innate tissues like hair can complicate evaluation and tissue management. The presence of soil contamination, which is common in equine wounds, can enhance the establishment of local sepsis. Typically, 10^6 microorganisms are required to cause bacterial infection. This inoculum can be reduced to 10^2 organisms in the presence of 5 mg of clay, the inorganic component of soil.[3] Early and appropriate cleansing and debridement can reduce potential healing delays. With chronicity, factors such as uncontrolled wound site movement and local sepsis can also delay and complicate healing. These factors should be considered on the initial examination.[4] Appropriate initial lavage can assist in removing contaminates, exudate, and other materials that complicate wound diagnostics. Guidance for lavage solution selection, volume, pressure, and other considerations are described in Karl E. Frees' article, "Equine Practice on Wound Management Wound: Cleansing and Hygiene," in this issue.

Investigating and noting the conformation of a wound is important to management decisions. This observation may be most pertinent to skin wounds, but the direction and extent of a wound should also be determined for deeper tissues. In skin, wound conformation can substantially influence vascularity, future blood flow and decisions on wound closure (see Louis Kamus and Christine Theoret's article, "Choosing the Best Approach to Wound Management and Closure," in this issue). For example, noting the conformation of a skin flap is very important. A skin flap with a proximally oriented broad base is much more amenable to successful closure with suture than the very common "inverted V" conformed flap. This inverted V is also often associated with tearing of skin versus sharp laceration, another consideration when regarding future vascular perfusion.

Puncture wounds can also present diagnostic challenges. Even discovering that a puncture through the skin has occurred can be difficult, as an obvious external wound may not be apparent. The presence of small volumes of blood, serum, or other fluid may be the only external sign over haired skin. Therefore, suspected puncture wound sites should have hair clipped such that the underlying skin can be investigated thoroughly. Manipulation, probing, and imaging may be required to gain a complete diagnosis of potential puncture wounds.

Another factor that should be noted is present and future motion of wounded tissues. The horse is an obligate weight bearer and will therefore typically use the wounded limb and place injured tissues in motion. The extent of limb motion at the time of initial wound management and throughout the time needed for healing should be carefully considered. Controlling motion can be a key to success in managing equine limb wounds and may require substantial external support. Appropriate use of bandages and rigid support are discussed in Randy B. Eggleston's article, "Equine Wound Management: Bandages, Casts, and External Support," in this issue.

Tissue loss is often a result of many equine distal limb wounding episodes. This occurrence is common with wounds from fence materials like barbed wire. Acute tissue loss can be obvious and occasionally can be subtle, with varying volumes of skin loss being most common. It is important to observe and note any loss of skin and other tissues, because wound management decisions are greatly influenced by this determination. Some tissue loss is delayed owing to vascular influences on torn tissue (skin) margins and occasionally secondary to crushing injury, which involves the local vasculature. Management decisions may need to be delayed several days while wounded tissue viability is completely delineated (**Figs. 2** and **3**).

MANIPULATIVE EXAMINATION

When deemed safe to perform, a manual palpation examination is indicated in the early diagnostic efforts for most equine limb wounds. Exceptions to prioritizing palpation would be the early need to more completely evaluate structural tissues via imaging techniques. Palpation and manipulation can cause air accumulation under wounded skin margins and potentially complicate imaging interpretations. To avoid this, discretion may indicate taking radiographs or performing an ultrasound examination before wound and deep tissue palpation. This strategy is especially true for suspected bone, ligament, tendon, tendon sheath, and joint involvement in a wound. Wounds that potentially involve a synovial compartment (ie, joint, tendon sheath, bursa) should be very closely evaluated, because delays in addressing potential or existing synovial sepsis can negatively influence future soundness and even survival. This issue is addressed in greater detail in Elsa K. Ludwig and Philip D. van Harreveld's article, "Equine Wounds over Synovial Structures," in this issue.

After appropriate initial wound cleansing (see Karl E. Frees' article, "Equine Practice on Wound Management: Wound Cleansing and Hygiene," in this issue), manual palpation can be very helpful in the diagnostic understanding of what tissues are injured. Sterile

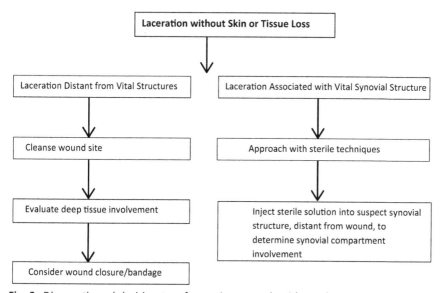

Fig. 2. Diagnostic and decision tree for equine wounds without skin or tissue loss.

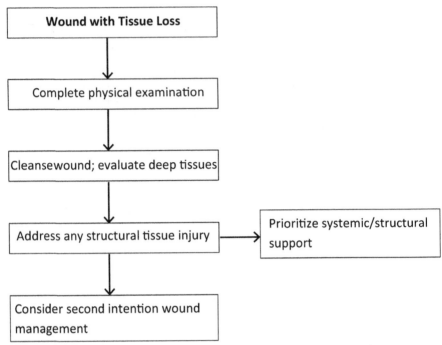

Fig. 3. Diagnostic and decision tree for equine wounds with skin or tissue loss.

gloves are recommended such that additional, inadvertent contamination is avoided. The tactile advantages of using fingers are hard to overemphasize. Careful tissue manipulation with fingers or with a sterile probe or forceps can reveal tissue disruption and also gauge the degree of deep contamination with foreign material. This examination can also occur while cleaning the wound site. As described in Karl E. Frees' article, "Equine Practice on Wound Management: Wound Cleansing and Hygiene," in this issue, it is important to avoid any additional harm to the wounded tissues. The selection of cleansing agents and techniques should be carefully determined.

Noting the cardinal signs of inflammation is important to gaining a complete understanding of a limb wound, as well as local and potential systemic repercussions. Heat, pain, and swelling are the most likely signs of inflammation to be present and the extent of these signs should be noted. Redness and capillary dilation are difficult to determine in dark pigmented and haired skin; however, these cardinal signs may be apparent in lightly colored, clipped regions. Lameness and/or reduction in normal weight bearing of an injured limb should also be noted and approached carefully in diagnostic efforts. Understanding the cardinal signs of inflammation in concert with other diagnostic results can enhance an understanding of the effects of a wound on a horse and limb.

RANGE OF MOTION EXAMINATION

Manipulation of an injured limb can also expose the depths of wound penetration. When the systemic physical examination and restraint indicate it is safe, a wounded limb can be picked up such that injured tissues can be observed through a passive range of motion exercise that can reveal more information than when a limb is in weight bearing. "Do no harm" should be the guiding principle.

EXAMINATION UNDER GENERAL ANESTHESIA

In some circumstances, a wound can be best evaluated with the affected horse under general anesthesia. This process can be safe if the horse is considered a stable candidate for anesthesia and the musculoskeletal and neurologic tissues are stable enough to support a safe and successful anesthetic recovery. If weight bearing support tissues are a concern, rigid external support may be required for safe anesthetic recovery (see Randy B. Eggleston's article, "Equine Wound Management: Bandages, Casts, and External Support," in this issue). Wound exploration and complete cleansing can be enhanced, and wound management more successfully initiated with a horse under general anesthesia. Removing a horse's avoidance responses and negative responses to painful stimuli allow more aggressive and thorough wound exploration. Although not often necessary, general anesthesia in the field with IV anesthetic drugs and/or in an operating room with IV or inhalant agents should be considered when safely possible.

DIAGNOSTIC INJECTION TECHNIQUES

Diagnostic injection techniques can be very helpful for complete wound assessment. This process is carefully reviewed in Elsa K. Ludwig and Philip D. van Harreveld's article, "Equine Wounds over Synovial Structures," in this issue in regard to potential synovial wounds. These techniques can also be helpful when synovial involvement is not suspected. The use of sterile, clear solutions (ie, saline, lactated Ringers) and vital stains, as well as the use of opaque, radiographic dyes (ie, iohexol) can assist diagnosis. With large surface wounds, wounds with widespread subcutaneous air presence, or with skin loss, these techniques are not very rewarding and perhaps should be avoided. The best return of diagnostic information is obtained when evaluating puncture wounds, wounds that may have foreign material in the deepest wounded tissue, or wounds that may enter a vital compartment (ie, synovial compartment; **Fig. 4**). A small exit portal, as seen with puncture wounds, likely allows the best information to be obtained. Survey radiographs are recommended before injection of any solution into a wound. This is due to the image altering capabilities of these liquid solutions, as well as accompanying air that is often injected with the chosen solution. Radiographic dyes and vital tissue stains can help to identify the depths a puncture wound may have reached, as well as outline the presence of foreign material. This finding can be helpful in acutely and chronically draining wounds with narrow or small exit wounds or fistulas. When a wound is considered to have potentially penetrated a synovial compartment, confirmation of suspected penetration can be determined with injection techniques. Injecting sterile, clear solutions into a suspected synovial compartment, distant from the wound, through intact, disinfected skin can make this diagnosis. It is important to maximally distend the compartment. If injected fluid egresses from the wound, joint, tendon sheath, or bursal penetration from the wound is confirmed. Distention of the synovial compartment without egress of the injected fluid strongly implies that the synovial compartment is intact and not wounded. In some unusual instances, suspect synovial compartments, having been assessed as intact, have become open and contaminated after tissue necrosis occurs 3 to 5 days after wounding. This secondary opening of a synovial space is likely due to latent vascular interruption to overlying tissues. Although not common, this phenomenon should be recognized as possible, especially with torn, potentially devitalized tissue associated with any suspect synovial compartment.

The use of these diagnostic injection techniques may need to be delayed or avoided if survey radiography indicates other management steps should take

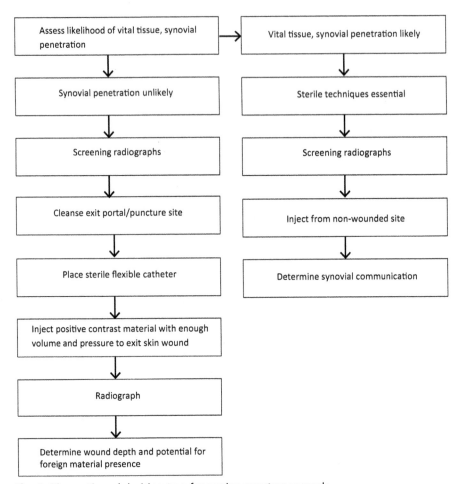

Fig. 4. Diagnostic and decision tree for equine puncture wounds.

priority. Radiographic evidence of bone injury, septic osteitis, and extensive dissection of air/gas warrant further investigation and probably prioritization of treatment protocols.

SUMMARY

A complete physical examination is indicated for any wounded horse. Systemic influences from a wound, like substantial hemorrhage, should be prioritized over wound management exercises to address any potential life threatening repercussions. However, most equine limb wounds are not life threatening and a direct wound evaluation can progress in a timely fashion. Visual, manipulative, and some invasive examination techniques should progress in a systematic manner such that all injured tissues are understood and treatment decisions can be made to maximize healing potential, decrease a horse's down time, and achieve the most satisfactory result possible.

REFERENCES

1. Peacock EE. Wound repair. 3rd edition. Philadelphia: WB Saunders, Co; 1984.

2. Robinson NE, Sprayberry KA. Current therapy in equine medicine. 6th edition. St Louis (MO): Saunders, Elsevier; 2009.
3. Caron JP. Management of superficial wounds. In: Auer JA, Stick JA, editors. Equine surgery. 2nd edition. Philadelphia: Saunders; 1999. p. 129–40.
4. Knottenbelt DC. Handbook of equine wound management. Edinburgh (Scotland): Saunders; 2003. p. 39–77.

Equine Practice on Wound Management
Wound Cleansing and Hygiene

Karl E. Frees, DVM, MS

KEYWORDS

- Equine • Wound management • Wound cleansing and hygiene • Healing

KEY POINTS

- The main goal of wound cleansing and care is the control or removal of tissue infection to allow healing to proceed efficiently.
- What should be kept in mind is that the benefit of a clean wound must be weighed against the trauma inflicted in the process of cleansing.
- Veterinarians and staff need to include the consistent practice of hand hygiene throughout the workday in order to reduce the chances of cross-contamination.

Wound management can be a daily occurrence, with the goals of therapy being restoration of function and an acceptable cosmetic outcome in the shortest amount of time and at the least cost possible. Achieving these goals often depends on control of infection and the reduction of deleterious effects on healing that local sepsis can create. Attempts to avoid infection and optimize wound healing begin at the initial assessment and the chosen approach to wound cleansing. Veterinarians have the potential to have a positive or negative influence, depending on wound cleansing and management as well as attention to personal hygiene. Local infection control and avoiding iatrogenic contamination are essential to good wound management.

A recent review pointed out that the World Health Organization (WHO) considers hand hygiene a pillar of infection control (particularly when related to nosocomial and iatrogenic infections), with a strong focus on their "Clean Hands Save Lives" campaign, which may translate into "Clean Hands Save Horses."[1] In the nineteenth century, human patient morbidity was substantially reduced with the recognition of germs/microorganisms (sepsis: the presence in tissues of harmful bacteria and their toxins, typically after entry from a wound), the introduction of hand hygiene (asepsis: preventing sepsis/working germ free from the start) and antiseptic principles (combating sepsis). Essentially, in the mid 1800s, it became clear that instead of just treating infections, the focus should be on prevention.

The author has no relationship with a commercial company to disclose.
Wilhite & Frees Equine Hospital, 21215 S. Peculiar Drive, Peculiar, MO 64078, USA
E-mail address: freesdvm@gmail.com

Vet Clin Equine 34 (2018) 473–484
https://doi.org/10.1016/j.cveq.2018.07.004
0749-0739/18/© 2018 Elsevier Inc. All rights reserved.

Skin has a balanced ecosystem of resident microbes, generally not pathogenic on intact skin, and transient microbes that are present via contact with patients, staff, and environmental surfaces. Resident microbes compete for nutrients with transient microbes, which are the most common cause of health care–associated infections (HAIs). Maintaining a positive balance to reduce transmission of pathogenic bacteria through hand hygiene is as important as is maintaining the natural skin environment and barrier. This task can be more difficult when working with equine patients because the environment can be rough on hands, leading to damage and irritation. Frequent contact with infected wounds and dirty environments creates a need for frequent hand washing. However, repeated hand washing can compromise skin integrity, lead to contact irritant dermatitis, and potentiate colonization with pathogenic microbes. Balance of hygiene and skin health is important.

- HAIs are often transferred from the hands of health care personnel to their patients.
  - Catheter site infections
  - Respiratory and urinary tract infections
  - Wound infections (inspections and bandage changes)
  - Hand hygiene is a simple and effective way to reduce HAIs
- The WHO guidelines (adapted by Verwilghen in 2016) on hand hygiene recommend 5 moments when caring for patients[2]:
  1. Before touching the patient
  2. Before a clean/aseptic procedure
  3. After body fluid exposure risk
  4. After touching the patient
  5. After touching patient surroundings
- Ways to support healthy skin
  1. Wash hands with a mild detergent soap when organic matter needs to be removed.
  2. Do not scrub hands in a manner that irritates skin.
  3. Use alcohol sanitizers for most hand cleaning, preferably with moisturizing ingredients.
  4. Use hand moisturizing lotion throughout the day to help protect skin barrier status.

WHAT IS THE RIGHT WAY TO WASH YOUR HANDS?

From the Centers for Disease Control and Prevention Web site: follow the 5 steps below to wash hands the right way every time[3]:

- *Wet* hands with clean, running water (warm or cold), turn off the tap, and apply soap.
- *Lather* hands by rubbing them together with the soap. Be sure to lather the backs of hands, between your fingers, and under your nails.
- *Rub* hands for at least 20 seconds.
- *Rinse* hands well under clean, running water.
- *Dry* hands using a clean towel or air dry them.

WHAT SHOULD YOU DO IF YOU DO NOT HAVE SOAP AND CLEAN, RUNNING WATER?

Washing hands with soap and water is the best way to get rid of microorganisms. If soap and water are not available, use an alcohol-based hand sanitizer that contains at least 60% alcohol. The product label can verify that the sanitizer contains at least 60%

alcohol. Alcohol-based hand sanitizers can quickly reduce the number of microorganisms on hands in some situations, but sanitizers do NOT get rid of all types of microorganisms. Hand sanitizers may not be as effective when hands are visibly dirty or greasy.

HOW DO YOU USE HAND SANITIZERS?

- Apply the gel to the palm of one hand (read the label to learn the correct amount).
- Rub hands together.
- Rub the gel over all surfaces of hands and fingers until hands are dry. This should take around 20 seconds.

Despite the benefits of hand hygiene against HAIs, including surgical site infections, septic processes in wounds remain a serious problem in human and veterinary medicine. In addition, there is the danger of zoonotic infections, including infection with methicillin-resistant *Staphylococcus aureus*, which can be a substantial concern between horses and humans.

WHAT IS THE PROPER WAY TO ENCOURAGE AND PRACTICE HAND HYGIENE?

- Recognize that skin health and integrity are important, so decontamination methods and products that are the least harmful to the skin are key.
  - Aggressive brushing or harsh disinfecting soaps are not indicated.
  - Sanitizing products with conditioners and emollients to support skin health are recommended.
  - Frequent application of skin care creams and lotions is recommended.
- When hands are visibly soiled with body fluids or other organic material, they should be washed with a gentle pH neutral nonmedicated soap.
- When not visibly soiled, an alcohol-based hand sanitizer should be used.
  - A product with 60% or greater ethyl alcohol should be used.
  - Ideally the product chosen would also contain hand conditioners, such as aloe and vitamin E.
- Compliance will be enhanced by ensuring the following:
  - Product accessibility, including soap, disposable towels, alcohol sanitizer, examination gloves, and skin care lotions.
    - Dispensers should be at several locations:
      - Sinks and other wash stations (**Fig. 1**)
      - Entrances to examination rooms, barn aisles, and stalls
      - On medicine and bandage carts
  - Staff education
    - Frequent reminders and examples
    - Handouts and posters

WOUND CLEANSING

Wound healing typically follows 3 phases: acute inflammation, repair (or proliferation), and maturation. When the acute response is too great or prolonged, transition into the repair phase can be delayed. The greatest ability to influence healing after wounding likely involves the acute inflammatory phase and initial wound management. Factors that influence the inflammatory response include the following:

- Severity and type of injury (such as sharp vs blunt trauma)
- Foreign material and devitalized tissue
- Infection

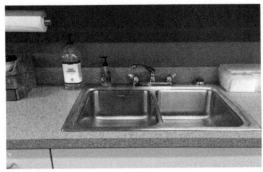

Fig. 1. Hand cleansing products: soap, alcohol sanitizer, and clean towels, should be readily accessible.

All open wounds contain bacteria, and potentially other microorganisms, that come from the environment or the horse. These bacteria can be contaminants (not replicating in the wound) of limited consequence; they can colonize (replicating but not causing trauma), or they can cause infection. Wound infection is established when enough microorganisms are present in a wound to cause host-tissue injury, generally accepted as when the number is greater than 10^6 bacteria per gram of tissue. The type of injury/wound sustained and the systemic condition of the horse influence the presence of a local septic process. Other factors that favor wound infection are as follows:

- Contamination with feces, which can contain 10^{11} bacteria per gram
- Contamination with soil, which can contain infection potentiating factors from organic or clay components
  - Infection can appear with as little as 100 microorganisms per gram
- The virulence of offending bacteria
- Reduced local defense mechanisms due to damaged blood supply, foreign body presence, or necrotic tissue

Initial wound cleansing can help reduce these adverse influences. "First do no harm" is an appropriate guiding principle. Attention to wound environment and veterinary hygiene is important. Good personal hygiene is especially important in challenging environments, such as paddocks, stalls, and barn aisles, and even hospitals with potential nosocomial pathogens and iatrogenic contamination.

SUGGESTED PREPARATIONS FOR INITIAL WOUND MANAGEMENT, AVOIDING FURTHER/CROSS-CONTAMINATION

- Use a clean, manageable work site with minimal disruptive traffic.
- Set up a clean area. Supplies can be securely placed on a portable table (**Fig. 2**).
- All commonly used supplies should be readily available.
- Grooming tools can be used to clean debris off the horse and the region of the wound.
  - A temporary bandage can cover a wound while brushing hair and debris from the surrounding area (**Fig. 3**).
- Wash hands and then use a hand sanitizer before donning examination gloves.
  - If soap and water are not available, an alcohol-based hand sanitizer (>60% ethyl alcohol) can be used alone.

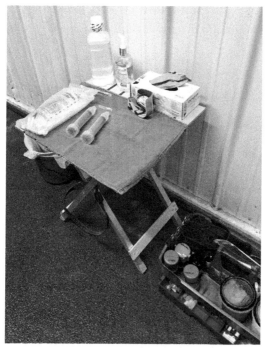

Fig. 2. Supplies can be kept clean and organized on a portable table.

- Clip hair from a large area starting at the edges of the wound and move outward a few inches in all directions (**Fig. 4**).
  - Clipper blades should be sharp and clean (disinfect between patients).
  - Wetting hair around the wound with water can reduce the potential for hair to fall into the wound while clipping.
  - Sterile, water-based lubricating gel can be placed into the wound OR gel-soaked gauze sponges can also be placed into the wound. These methods also retard entry of hair and debris into a wound.
- Sanitize hands again and don fresh gloves before proceeding to further address the wound.

CLEANSE THE WOUND

It is impossible to completely eliminate bacteria from a wound. The goal of cleansing is to reduce the volume of necrotic debris and bacterial numbers. It is important to realize that any form of cleaning, mechanical (scrubbing with gauze) or chemical (antiseptic agents), will involve some level of debridement to remove contamination and devitalized tissue. In some cases, the physical damage and cytotoxicity are more traumatic to the wound than they may be beneficial. Therefore, the form and force of cleaning should be balanced between the desired effect and potential for harm to the tissue.

SCRUBBING/PHYSICAL CLEANSING

- In the past, "scrubbing" the wound was the most common form of physical debridement used and is one of the most effective and rapid means of reducing

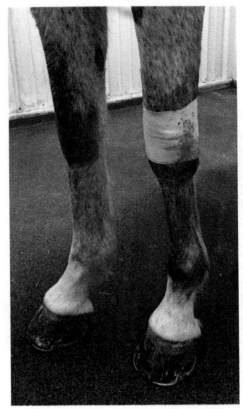

Fig. 3. A temporary bandage in place to cover and protect the wound while the rest of the limb is brushed off.

the bacterial load in a wound. However, physical scrubbing is nonselective and may delay wound healing by damaging normal tissue. Generally, scrubbing should be limited to the intact skin around the wound, and any application of force to wounded tissue should be limited to the least amount possible to achieve wound decontamination (**Fig. 5**). A study on intact skin of horses compared 5 minutes of mechanical scrubbing with gauze sponges and 4% chlorhexidine gluconate detergent (CH) to a second group where CH and sponges were used for 15 seconds to attain a lather, which was left for just more than 4 minutes skin contact time. The reduced mechanical scrubbing technique was as effective in reducing bacterial numbers on the skin as the traditional 5-minute scrub.[4]

- Usually performed by "scrubbing" with gauze (woven gauze is more abrasive than nonwoven).
- Recognize that desired superficial fibroblasts and epithelial cells will be removed along with deleterious contamination.
- Use the least amount of force and least abrasive technique possible to remove soil, feces, devitalized tissue, and other contaminants.
- Use of the sponge portion (not the bristles) of a surgical scrub brush, especially when moistened, can be used as a lower friction cleaning tool.
- The scrubbed area can be rinsed with sponges soaked in sterile saline or with 70% isopropyl alcohol (intact skin only). Larger areas can be rinsed by

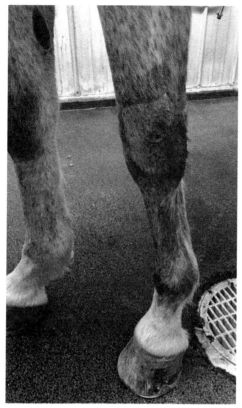

Fig. 4. Clip hair around the wound in a perimeter large enough to allow proper cleansing. The surrounding hair can be wetted, and sterile gel can be placed in the wound to reduce the entry of hair and debris into the wound.

puncturing 3 to 4 holes in the top of a 1-L bottle of saline with a 14-gauge needle (**Fig. 6**A) and using it as a squeeze bottle (**Fig. 6**B).

ANTISEPTICS

- Antiseptic agents have been used for skin preparation, wound cleaning, and lavage. Although topical antiseptics will reduce the bacterial load in wounded tissue, they are nonselectively cytotoxic and will damage all cell types on contact. Because of their cellular toxicity their use, and that of isopropyl alcohol, is best limited to intact tissue around a wound.[5]
  - Povidone iodine (PI) has a broad spectrum of activity against gram-positive and gram-negative bacteria and fungi. Its use is best limited to intact peri-wound tissues.
  - CH has a broad antimicrobial spectrum of activity that has a residual effect due to its binding to the stratum corneum of skin. CH is contraindicated around the cornea and open synovial structures, and use is best limited to intact peri-wound tissues.
  - Prior studies in humans and animals have not found clear evidence to favor one antiseptic over another, what seems to be generally agreed upon is to avoid open wound contact with antiseptics or alcohol.

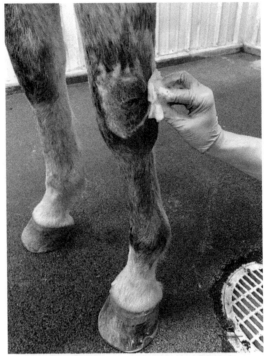

Fig. 5. Scrubbing and the use of antiseptics should be limited to the intact periwound tissue.

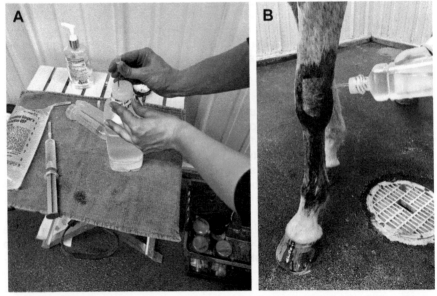

Fig. 6. (*A*) A needle can be used to puncture the top of a bottle of saline for rinsing of larger areas. (*B*) Using a squeeze bottle of saline for rinsing.

○ Hydrogen peroxide, acetic acid (distilled vinegar), and Dakin solution (0.5% solution of sodium hypochlorite/bleach) are other occasionally mentioned antiseptics; the balance between the positive and negative effects of their use may be more difficult to determine, and so their use is left to the careful discrimination of the operator.

WOUND LAVAGE

- Hydrotherapy can be effective in reducing contamination of a wound while being less damaging than scrubbing and antiseptics to normal tissue. Irrigation should be the mainstay of wound-cleansing techniques.
  ○ In a fresh wound (<3 hours old, minimal inflammatory response), adequate cleaning can be accomplished with just water or a sterile isotonic fluid like normal saline (0.9% NaCl) or lactated Ringer solution (LRS). Wounds of longer duration, in which bacteria become more established, will most likely require some level of careful debridement.
  ○ Irrigation technique
    ■ To overcome the adherence of bacteria to a wound while avoiding tissue damage or driving bacteria deeper into tissues, the fluid should be delivered at a pressure of 8 to 15 psi.[6] The stream should be at an oblique angle to the surface of the wound (**Fig. 7**).
      • Approximately 15 psi pressure can be achieved using a 35-mL syringe and a 19-gauge needle.[7]
      • Commercial irrigation systems are available, such as the Interpulse System (Stryker, Kalamazoo, MI, USA) and the Sidekick Water Flosser (Waterpik, Inc, Fort Collins, CO, USA).
  ○ Irrigation fluid selection
    ■ Isotonic fluids, such as normal saline or LRS, will provide an irrigation medium that is least harmful to the wounded tissue.
    ■ If greater volumes are needed for larger or multiple wounds, tap water can be initially used to produce "homemade saline."
      • Saline solution can be made by adding 8 teaspoons of salt to 1 gallon of boiled water (or 2 teaspoons [10 mL] of salt per liter) and then cooled.
      • For larger irrigation volumes, a 1-gallon "garden sprayer" can be used (purchased for dedicated wound use). To gauge proper pressure, approximate the feel of the stream from a home shower and maintain a distance of at least 6 inches from the sprayer tip to the wound (**Fig. 8**).
  ○ Although there are no guidelines to govern total volume of irrigation fluid, an amount that removes visible debris and contamination without causing the tissue to become swollen or blanched (waterlogged) is recommended.
  ○ Although cleansing an acute wound is often safely accomplished using saline or LRS, chronic or heavily contaminated wounds may benefit from the addition of an antiseptic (to a diluted level) in an effort to reduce the expected bacterial load of the wound. Debate, regarding what additives to use, continues as results of conflicting studies (in vitro vs in vivo findings) can be difficult to interpret and put to clinical use for the horse.
    ■ Use of antiseptics like PI and CH in diluted form will allow a balance between antimicrobial action and tissue cytotoxicity.[5]
      • PI 10% solution can be diluted to a concentration of 0.1% by adding 10 mL per liter of irrigation fluid.
      • CH 2% solution can be diluted to a concentration of 0.05% by adding 25 mL per 975 mL of irrigation fluid.

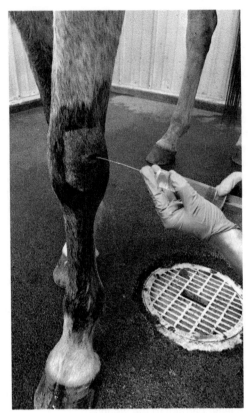

Fig. 7. A syringe and needle can be used to apply irrigation cleansing and gentle debridement to the wound.

- Use of antibiotics as additives to lavage fluid should be discouraged or only approached with due caution regarding concerns of developing bacterial resistance.

REPEATED WOUND CLEANSING

Serial wound cleansing may be needed in heavily contaminated wounds and those healing by second intention to remove substances deleterious to the healing process, such as organic debris, exudate, and necrotic tissue.

- Approach each repeat wound examination and cleansing session with the same care as the initial examination. The balance between the force of cleaning and materials used to benefit the healing wound, against the potential deleterious effects on the tissue and propagating cells (epithelial cells and fibroblasts), becomes very important in making decisions.
  - Practice proper hand hygiene.
  - Clean off gross debris from the horse.
  - Repeat hand hygiene.
  - Remove the bandage and visually inspect the wound.
  - Repeat hand hygiene and don gloves.
  - Address the wound as needed.

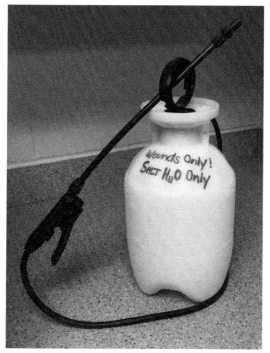

Fig. 8. For very large wounds or multiple wounds that require large volumes of irrigation fluid, a garden sprayer can be purchased and dedicated for wound lavage.

- ○ Repeat hand hygiene.
- ○ Reapply dressing and a bandage if indicated.
- ○ Repeat hand hygiene.

The main goal of wound cleansing and care is the control or removal of tissue infection to allow healing to proceed in the most functional, cosmetic, fastest, and least expensive manner possible. These attempts at decontamination are accomplished through the removal of debris and necrotic tissue while reducing the bacterial load via careful use of mechanical techniques and cleaning agents, accepting that some level of tissue trauma will result. What must always be kept in mind is that the benefit of a clean wound must be weighed against the trauma inflicted in the process of cleansing. In addition, it must be realized that veterinarians and staff need to include the consistent practice of hand hygiene throughout the workday in order to reduce the chances of cross-contamination to equine patients and also transfer of zoonotic pathogens to humans. Veterinary health care professionals should constantly be taking steps to reduce the incidence of hospital-acquired infections and zoonotic disease transmission. Although the condition in which patients are presented cannot be controlled, human impact, negative and otherwise, on the patient's health can be controlled.

REFERENCES

1. Verwilghen D. The World Health Organization's Clean Hands Save Lives: a concept applicable to equine medicine as Clean Hands Save Horses. Equine Vet Educ 2016 [early view: 1–9]. [Epub ahead of print].

2. Supplement to Reference 1. https://onlinelibrary.wiley.com/action/download Supplement?doi=10.1111%2Feve.12680&file=eve12680-sup-0002-ItemS2.pdf
3. Centers for Disease Control and Prevention. Wash your hands. 2018. Available at: https://www.cdc.gov/features/handwashing/index.html. Accessed June 2018.
4. Davids BI, Davidson MJ, TenBroeck SH, et al. Efficacy of mechanical versus non-mechanical sterile preoperative skin preparation with chlorhexidine gluconate 4 % solution. Vet Surg 2015;44:648.
5. Rani SA, Hoon R, Najafi RR, et al. The *in vitro* antimicrobial activity of wound and skin cleansers at nontoxic concentrations. Adv Skin Wound Care 2014;27:65.
6. Barnes S, Spencer M, Graham D, et al. Surgical wound irrigation: a call for evidence-based standardization of practice. Am J Infect Control 2014;42:525.
7. Singer A, Hollander J, Subramanian S, et al. Pressure dynamics of various irrigation techniques commonly used in the emergency department. Ann Emerg Med 1994;1:36.

Topical Wound Medications

Britta S. Leise, DVM, PhD

KEYWORDS

- Horse • Wound healing • Ointments • Antiseptics • Topical antimicrobials

KEY POINTS

- Topical antiseptics used for wound cleansing should be diluted appropriately to maximize microbial killing and minimize cytotoxic effects to the wound bed.
- When possible, topical antimicrobial medications are recommended in place of systemic antibiotics in the management of equine wounds. Topical antimicrobials can be more effective, because many have the ability to work in the presence of a biofilm or have properties to help eliminate biofilms from the wound bed.
- Topical medications can be used to manipulate the healing process or enhance the wound environment to promote healing. For example, corticosteroids can be used when excessive granulation tissue is present. Other therapies, such as honey or platelet-rich plasma, have various properties that improve autolytic débridement of wounds and provide factors that improve normal wound healing.

LAVAGE SOLUTIONS

Topical cleaning agents should provide antisepsis but should not be cytotoxic to the healthy tissue within a wound. Prior to antiseptic application, a wound should be prepared by applying a water-soluble sterile lubricant, followed by clipping of the wound margins to remove hair. Many equine wounds have substantial contamination with dirt and debris and may have been cleaned by a layperson prior to the arrival of the veterinarian. In these cases, nonsterile tap water may have been used. Although irrigating wounds with tap water does not increase microbial colonization,[1] the use of tap water is reported to be cytotoxic to skin fibroblasts.[2] The cytotoxic effects of tap water are attributed to alkaline pH, hypotonicity, and presence of cytotoxic trace elements.[2] Clinically, however, in humans the use of tap water to clean wound does not delay healing.

The most common agent used by veterinarians to clean equine wounds is 0.9% sodium chloride. Saline provides its antiseptic effects via dilution when used as a lavage. Saline, however, does have mild cytotoxic effects in vitro on canine fibroblasts after 10 minutes of exposure. This results from the slightly acidic pH of normal saline and the lack of a buffering system. Lactated Ringer solution does not result in fibroblast damage[2]; therefore, the use of such isotonic solutions may be preferred over the use of 0.9% sodium chloride.

Disclosure Statement: The author has nothing to disclose.
Equine Surgery, Veterinary Clinical Sciences, Louisiana State University, School of Veterinary Medicine, Skip Bertman Drive, Baton Rouge, LA 70803, USA
E-mail address: bleise@lsu.edu

Vet Clin Equine 34 (2018) 485–498
https://doi.org/10.1016/j.cveq.2018.07.006
0749-0739/18/Published by Elsevier Inc.
vetequine.theclinics.com

Removal of dirt and debris from the wound is important, because soil has been found to have factors that potentiate infection. In the presence of soil, only 100 bacteria are necessary to elicit infection.[3] Therefore, topical cleansing of wounds is an important part of wound management. Pressure lavage can be used to help clean and decontaminate wounds; however, it is important not to be too aggressive. Lavage pressures over 20 psi can damage tissue and drive bacteria deeper into a wound bed. Use of a 35-mL syringe with a 19-gauge needle exerts a pressure of 7 psi to 15 psi at a wound surface (**Fig. 1**).[3,4] Additional cleansing of the wound after the initial treatment may be unnecessary, because it may damage the delicate tissue around the wound margin and remove wound exudate that can have beneficial factors for wound healing.

ANTISEPTICS

Antiseptics can be used alone or added to lavage fluid to reduce microbial content within a wound (**Fig. 2**). Topical antiseptics should have a broad spectrum of activity, controlling both resident and contaminating flora, including bacteria, fungi, and viruses on the wound and surrounding skin. Antiseptics reduce microbial numbers through mechanical and/or chemical properties. The addition of antiseptics, such as povidone-iodine or chlorhexidine, into lavage fluid is a common practice in equine wound management. It is important, however, to dilute these products to appropriate levels (0.1%–0.05% solutions) that minimize deleterious effects to the wound and surrounding tissue prior to use, because many of these antiseptic agents have negative effects on wound healing at higher concentrations.

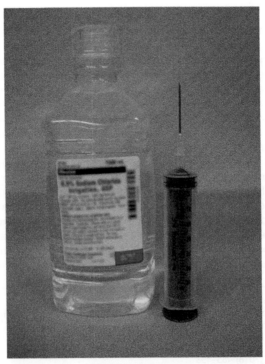

Fig. 1. Normal saline (0.9% sodium chloride) administered as a pressure lavage using an 18-gauge needle and 35-mL syringe will deliver between 8 psi and 15 psi to the wound surface.

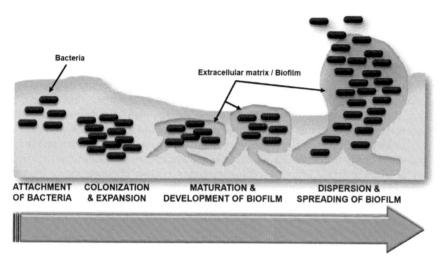

Fig. 2. Development of a biofilm occurs when microorganisms (purple) colonize into communities on the surface of wounds, producing a protective extracellular matrix (green) that encases the organisms, preventing antimicrobial penetration.

Hydrogen Peroxide 3%

Hydrogen peroxide 3% is used to clean wounds, producing an effervescent effect on application. The antimicrobial benefits of hydrogen peroxide in vivo have been questioned because it is rapidly broken down into water and oxygen, via the enzyme catalase, on contact with organic tissue. Bacterial production of catalyze likely limits the microbial killing ability of hydrogen peroxide. Due to its liberation of oxygen, hydrogen peroxide has been recommended for use in deep puncture wounds where *Clostridium* infections may be of concern. Numerous studies suggest that hydrogen peroxide is cytotoxic. Therefore, it is not recommended for use in the general cleaning of equine wounds. Use of a hydrogen peroxide cream has demonstrated improved healing of equine wounds. Experimentally, application of 1% hydrogen peroxide cream (LHP, Bioglan AB, Malmö, Sweden) resulted in faster healing of equine wounds and reduced bacterial colonization compared with controls.[5]

Povidone-Iodine 10%

Povidone-iodine is an iodophor and depends on the release of free iodine to be activated.[3,6] Iodophors were developed to stabilize iodine in solution and subsequently allow the sustained release of iodine. The antimicrobial action of povidone-iodine occurs rapidly, killing a variety of bacterial strains within 20 seconds to 30 seconds. Although the mechanism of action has not been fully elucidated, iodine damages essential cellular structures by attacking intracellular proteins, fatty acids, and nucleotides.[6] Iodine is inactivated by organic material; therefore, removal of dirt and debris is indicated prior to application of povidone-iodine. Prolonged microbial killing is also inhibited by the presence of organic material, such as blood and serum proteins, and effects on microbial killing is short lived. Povidone-iodine reportedly increased damage to vascular endothelium and caused thrombosis in rat wounds compared with other agents, including chlorhexidine.[7] Epithelialization can also be delayed when povidone-iodine is used.[6] Therefore, 10% povidone-iodine should be diluted to concentrations of 0.1% to 0.2% to minimize cytotoxicity to the surrounding tissue. The addition of 10 mL to 20 mL in 1 L of saline is recommend for cleaning equine wounds. It is important that scrub formulations are not used to clean wounds because the detergent component has increased cytotoxic effects on exposed tissues.

Chlorhexidine Gluconate and Chlorhexidine Diacetate 2%

Chlorhexidine is one of the most commonly used antiseptics in veterinary medicine. It is a biguanide antiseptic that is positively charged and exerts its antimicrobial effects by reacting with the negative cell surface membrane, thereby disrupting and subsequently killing microorganisms. It has a wide antimicrobial spectrum and a prolonged residual effect. Unlike povidone-iodine, the presence of organic material has no effect on the microbial killing ability of chlorhexidine. Bacterial resistance has developed through activation of efflux pumps, which are intermembrane protein channels developed by bacteria to remove various antibiotics and biocides. In particular, some *Pseudomonas* and *Proteus* spp have been found resistant to chlorhexidine.[8] Chlorhexidine can be cytotoxic; therefore, it must be diluted prior to use. A 0.05% solution is recommended for lavage and cleaning of wounds. A 1:40 dilution of chlorhexidine gluconate 2% can be made by adding 25 mL of 2% chlorhexidine to 975 mL of sterile saline. Chlorhexidine should not be used near the eye or open joints, as its use can result in corneal edema and scaring, affecting vision and synovial inflammation and abundant fibrin accumulation, respectively.[9] Overall, chlorhexidine is recommended for use over povidone-iodine, because it is less cytotoxic and has superior bacterial killing.

Dakin's Solution

Dakin's solution or sodium hypochlorite, also known as bleach, is available in varying concentrations ranging from full strength at 0.5% to 1/40 strength of 0.0125%. Sodium hypochlorite exerts its antibacterial effects by liberating chlorine into the tissues. Although bleach has been historically used to clean wounds in battlefield situations, Dakin's solution is cytotoxic; therefore, low dilutions (1:50 dilution resulting in 0.00025% solution) of the 0.0125% concentration are recommended. This solution is not stable and is inactivated by light and heat. Due to the instability and cytotoxic properties, sodium hypochlorite is not commonly used or recommended to treat equine wounds.

Hypochlorous Acid

Similar to hypochlorite, hypochlorous acid exerts its antimicrobial effects through the actions of chloride. Improved microbial killing occurs, however, when chlorine is in the presence of a solution with a low pH (5–6). This makes hypochlorous acid effective as an antiseptic and it is reported be 70 to 80 times more effective than hypochlorite for inactivating bacteria. In evaluation of 19 skin cleansers, hypochlorous acid had minimal cytotoxic effects and demonstrated the most rapid bacterial kill, with various commercial hypochlorous acid products. Application times have ranged between 1 minute to 30 minutes.[10] Although hypochlorous acid has been reported in vitro to achieve bacterial killing within biofilms, the actual biofilm structure was not disrupted by treatment.[11] This suggests that mechanical disruption of the biofilm (see **Fig. 2**) may be necessary when hypochlorous acid is used to treat chronic wounds.

Vetericyn (Innovacyn, Rialto, California) is a commercially available veterinary compound sold in 2 concentrations: (1) as an over-the-counter solution for horse owners and (2) as a veterinarian prescribed solution. The veterinary prescribed compound is comprised of 0.003% hypochlorous acid and 0.004% sodium hypochlorite. It is made by electrochemically treating water resulting in a hypochlorous solution with a neutral pH.[12] Processing has made this product stable, with an average shelf life of 24 months. Vetercyn is supplied as a ready-to-use solution and can be sprayed directly on wounds.

The combination of low cytotoxicity and rapid decontamination of bacteria makes hypochlorous acid a desirable antiseptic. Indications for use include initial wound cleaning of the acute injury and for daily cleaning of chronic wounds.

Tris–Ethylenediaminetetraacetic Acid

The combination of Tris buffer (tris[hydroxymethyl]aminomethane) and disodium-calcium salt of ethylenediaminetetraacetic acid (EDTA) results in microbial death after topical application, particularly to gram-negative bacteria, by increasing microbial cell membrane permeability. Although wounds with reduced pH levels have been associated with improvement in wound healing,[13] some antibiotics, such as aminoglycoside, do not perform well in an acidic environment. Tris-EDTA can be used to alkalize the surrounding tissue environment. This alkalization improves the function of some topically administered antibiotics, such as aminoglycoside. The increase in cell permeability and alkalization of the wound bed further allows Tris-ETDA to potentiate the bactericidal activity of many antibiotics, including aminoglycides, penicillin, and oxytetracycline.[14] Tris-EDTA also has the ability to disrupt biofilms. This disruption results from the chelation of the divalent cations, calcium and iron, by Tris-EDTA, causing bacterial cell detachment, lysis, and destabilization of biofilm.[15] Clinical uses involve the treatment of wounds infected with 4 major bacteria: *Pseudomonas aeruginosa*, *Staphylococcus aureus*, *Proteus vulgaris*, and *Escherichia coli*.[16]

The addition of 0.01% chlorhexidine to Tris-EDTA has been reported to have synergistic effects on microbial killing.[16] Although not commonly used to treat equine wounds, Tris-ETDA has been used in the management of uterine and sinus infections in horses. Indications for use in the horse include lavage solutions for penetrating wounds and fistulous tracts, both with and without the addition of antibiotics. Preparation of a Tris-EDTA solution has been described[16] and can be made from 1.2 g of EDTA and 6.05 of Tris buffer added to 1 L of sterile water (**Box 1**). The pH should be adjusted to 8.0 by adding dilute sodium hydroxide. After it is prepared, the Tris-EDTA solution should be autoclaved for 15 minutes.

Commercial Wound Cleansers

Due to environmental factors, equine wounds are frequently contaminated, resulting in the development of a biofilm that can delay wound healing. Cultures from both acute and chronic equine wounds have isolated multiple bacterial species with varying ability to develop biofilms. Bacterial biofilm formation allows for promotion of antimicrobial resistance and prevents the host immune system from eliciting a productive response.[17] Due to the addition of surfactants, some commercial wound cleansers can help treat bacterial contamination within a biofilm. Shur-Clens (ConvaTec, Oklahoma City, Oklahoma) is a wound cleanser that contains the nontoxic surfactant poloxamer 188.

Box 1
Common antiseptic preparations used in the management of equine wounds

- Povidone-iodine (0.1%–0.2%): povidone-iodine should be diluted to concentrations of 0.1%–0.2% to minimize cytotoxicity. This can be achieved by the addition of 10 mL to 20 mL of povidone iodine into 1 L of sterile saline.

- Chlorhexidine 0.05%: chlorhexidine should be diluted to concentrations of 0.05% to minimize cytotoxicity. This can be achieved by the addition of 25 mL of 2% chlorhexidine gluconate to 975 mL of sterile saline.

- Tris-EDTA: 1.2 g of EDTA and 6.05 of Tris added to 1 L of sterile water. The resulting solution should have a pH = 8.0 and undergo sterilization in the autoclave for 15 minutes.

Mechanical breakdown of biofilm occurs with this product; however, it has been recommended that it be used in conjunction with an antimicrobial agent, because poloxamer alone has no antimicrobial effects.

Many cleansers used for cleaning intact skin, such as shampoos and scrubs (including povidone-iodine and chlorhexidine scrubs), have cytotoxic properties to exposed tissues in wounds and should be avoided.

TOPICAL ANTIMICROBIALS

Topical antimicrobial agents can be useful when treating acute contaminated wounds and when managing chronic granulating wounds. Judicious use of systemic antibiotics for the treatment of equine wounds is strongly recommended, because antimicrobial resistance continues to rise. Many chronic granulating wounds develop a superficial biofilm that can delay healing (see **Fig. 2**; **Fig. 3**). Topical antimicrobials are aimed at treating the local environment and many are efficacious in the presence of a biofilm where systemic antibiotics would have little to no effect. Although some ointments can affect tissue microcirculation and perfusion,[18] their benefits can outweigh the potential negative effects and, in some cases, actually improve wound healing.

Triple Antibiotic Ointment

One of the classic topical antimicrobials used in both humans and animals is triple antibiotic ointment. It is comprised of 3 different antibiotics: neomycin, polymyxin B, and bacitracin. Triple antibiotic ointment has a wide antimicrobial spectrum, but it is ineffective against *Pseudomonas* spp. In people, the use of triple antibiotic ointment results in faster wound healing, reduces the number of colonizing bacteria, and decreases scarring. The zinc compound within the bacitracin component has been reported to

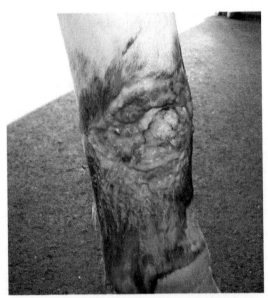

Fig. 3. Wire laceration of 10 days duration. Heavy bacterial colonization and presence of a biofilm is demonstrated by the presence of exudate. Use of topical cleansers with a noncytotoxic antiseptic is indicated in the treatment of this wound followed by the application of a topical antimicrobial.

stimulate epithelialization but may retard wound contraction. In horses, triple antibiotic ointment has been demonstrated to delay wound healing in the distal limb.[19] The mechanism for the delayed healing is believed associated with the petroleum base within the ointment, which can decrease epithelial proliferation. Regardless, the results from this study suggest that other topical therapies may have improved benefits over triple antibiotic ointment, and alternatives should be considered.[19]

Silver Sulfadiazine

Silver sulfadiazine (SSD) 1% ointment is a commonly used topical antibacterial agent for prevention of infection in burn wounds. SSD has a wide antimicrobial spectrum, including both gram-positive and gram-negative bacteria and fungi. Both the silver and sulfa antibiotic components of SSD interact with each other to provide antimicrobial effects. Silver binds to the microbes' DNA releasing of the sulfonamide, which inhibits metabolic pathways within the organism, thereby resulting in microbial death. SSD ointment has been the most effective agent evaluated when treating a multidrug-resistant *P aeruginosa* in full-thickness burn wounds.[20] Although no differences between povidone-iodine and SSD in the healing of distal limb wounds of horses have been identified, the antimicrobial properties of SSD could justify its use in contaminated wounds.[21] SSD should be applied under a light bandage, because it does not adhere well to equine wounds.[12] SSD should also be applied daily, because the silver ions can quickly become inactive once they react with wounded tissue.[12]

Sugar

Antimicrobial effects of granulated sugar on wounds result from the hyperosmolarity of this compound. Other hyperosmolar effects of sugar include wound débridement and a decrease in wound edema, as fluid is drawn out of the wound on application. Sugar is best applied during the early débridement and inflammatory stages of wound healing. It is indicated for use in highly exudative wounds and should be discontinued when a healthy bed of granulation tissue appears.[12] The addition of povidone-iodine to sugar creates a product known as sugardine. This product is commonly used in the treatment of hoof abscesses. Care should be taken when povidone-iodine is added to sugar because high concentrations of iodine can be cytotoxic.

Honey

Although honey has been used to treat wounds for centuries, recent studies have evaluated its effects on equine wounds. In general, honey has several antimicrobial properties. It is hyperosmolar and draws out fluid not only from microbes resulting in desiccation and death but also from the subcutaneous tissue to the wound surface, assisting in removal of debris and necrotic tissue and reducing edema. Honey contains an enzyme that catalyzes the production of hydrogen peroxide in low amounts resulting in microbial death. Manuka honey contains the antibacterial compound methylglyoxal, also known as Unique Manuka Factor (UMF).[22] The antimicrobial effects of Manuka honey are expressed by UMF with higher values demonstrating improved activity. When compared in equine distal limb wounds, Manuka honey with a UMF of 20 was superior in wound healing time compared with honey with a UMF of 5.[23]

Bischofberger and coworkers[24] evaluated the effects of Manuka honey on second intention wound healing in the distal limb of horses and observed that wounds treated with Manuka honey gel healed significantly faster than other wounds (both treated and nontreated) in their study. On average, wounds treated with Manuka honey healed 12 days faster than untreated wounds.[24] Various honey products have been evaluated; however, not all honey is created equal. Veterinarians have suggested that local produced honey may have improved antimicrobial benefits against resident bacteria versus medical grade honey. Evaluation of different honeys, including locally produced, medical-grade, and store-processed, found that 18 of 29 honeys had positive bacterial or fungal growth before exposure to bacterial isolates from wounds.[25] Nonmedical and processed honeys were more likely to have bacterial contamination. Therefore, the use of locally produced or store-bought honeys for the treatment of wounds may result in inadvertent contamination and are not recommend for wound therapy. When evaluated for their antimicrobial effectiveness on common equine wound isolates, Manuka honey (both medical-grade and store-bought) and heather honey (from a local bee producer) performed best, effectively killing all 10 bacterial isolates studied.[25] Honeys in this study were also compared with sugar solutions of that inhibited bacterial growth of only 5 of the 10 isolates tested.[25] Manuka honey gel (Medihoney, Derma Sciences, Plainsboro, New Jersey) can help decrease the cost of treatment, by eliminating the need for bandaging to keep the medication in contact with the wound. The use of honey seems to have the greatest impact on wound healing during the inflammatory and débridement stages; therefore, it is recommended for use during the first 2 to 3 weeks of wound healing.

Cadexomer Iodine

Cadexomer iodine, a more recently formulated iodophor product, was developed in the 1980s as an antiseptic agent. It is composed of 0.9% iodine mixed with a starch polymer bead that immobilizes the iodine molecules. Once the cadexomer iodine contacts the wound exudate, the polymer bead swells and gradually releases iodine molecules. The slow release of iodine, in cadexomer iodine, provides enhanced microbial killing compared with povidone-iodine. Cadexomer iodine was useful in treating MRSA and *Pseudomonas* infections when present as a biofilm in mice wounds.[26] Cadexomer has also been reported to increase production of proinflammatory mediators and vascular endothelial growth factor by macrophages. This activity can improve wound healing and enhance epithelization in full-thickness wounds.[27] Iodosorb Gel (Smith & Nephew, St. Petersburg, Florida), is a commercially available cadexomer product that can be applied topically to wounds. Although there are no reports of its use in horses, this product may be beneficial in the treatment of contaminated wounds.

Octenidine Wound Gel

Octenidine dihydrochloride is a cationic surfactant and pyridine derivative that was developed in the late 1980s as an antiseptic agent. It has a broad antimicrobial spectrum, including gram-positive and gram-negative bacteria and fungi. It has prolonged activity on skin and has been reported to be present up to 24 hours after application.[12] Octenidine has also demonstrated excellent efficacy for treatment of *P aeruginosa* and *S aureus* infections within biofilms.[8] Treatment of chronic venous leg ulcers in people found that application of an octenidine-based gel resulted in greater wound size reduction and faster healing.[28] Additionally, application of the gel alone had similar results with lower treatment costs, because bandaging was not necessary to have a beneficial effect.[28] Although this compound has not been tested in the horse, it may have several beneficial properties that warrant its use in the treatment of chronic wounds.

Nitrofurazone

Nitrofurazone is an inexpensive broad-spectrum antimicrobial with primary bacteriostatic effects. It is not effective against *Pseudomonas* spp and wound exudate reduces its potency. Nitrofurazone is available over the counter for owners and farm managers as an ointment. Nitrofurazone can decrease epithelialization and delay wound contraction in horses.[29] It is also believed to promote exuberant granulation tissue formation; therefore, it is not recommended to be placed on distal limb wounds. Nitrofurazone has been reported to cause ovarian and mammary tumors in rodents and suspected as carcinogenic to humans[30]; therefore, it is no longer allowed to be used in food producing animals.[12] Due to its limited antimicrobial activity and potential negative effects in equine wounds, other topical antimicrobials should be preferentially considered.

MANAGEMENT OF EXUBERANT GRANULATION TISSUE
Corticosteroids

The most common topical corticosteroid used in the treatment of equine wounds is triamcinolone used in combination with the antifungal nystatin and the antibiotics neomycin and thiostrepton (Animax (Dechra, Overland Park, KS) or Panalog (Fort Dodge Animal Health, Fort Dodge, IA)). Triamcinolone can suppress the early formation of exuberant granulation tissue in distal limb wounds of horses healing via second intention.[31] The exact mechanism by which corticosteroids decrease the production of exuberant granulation tissue is not known, but is it suspected to be related to a decrease in production of transforming growth factor β1 by monocytes and macrophages.[29] Judicious use of products containing triamcinolone is indicated because negative effects on wound healing are well documented with the use of steroids. Corticosteroids can substantially delay wound contraction, epithelialization, and angiogenesis.[32]

Topical corticosteroids can be beneficial in preparing a wound bed for skin grafting (**Box 2**). It is important, however, that the steroid be discontinued for a minimum of 3 days to 5 days before grafting occurs or success is negatively affected. Corticosteroids are contraindicated in the treatment of infected wounds because the host immune response is dampened, resulting in a decreased ability for the white blood cells to remove bacteria. Care also should be taken when treating extremely large wounds, because systemic absorption of triamcinolone can occur. Although uncommon, high doses of steroids, in particular triamcinolone (40–80 mg), and frequently repeated doses (of 15–20 mg/d of triamcinolone) over days to weeks have been reported to result in laminitis.[33] Although triamcinolone used topically should not be a concern in most horses, those with equine metabolic syndrome and/or pituitary pars intermedia dysfunction may have an increased risk of developing laminitis when large amounts are administered.

Granulex

Granulex is a topical compound comprised of trypsin, balsam of Peru, and castor oil. All 3 ingredients are believed to have an effect on wound healing, particularly in the

---

Box 2
Preparation of granulated wound bed for skin grafting using corticosteroids

1. Surgically débride the exuberant granulation tissue.

2. Topically apply the corticosteroid 2 days to 3 days post-débridement (only if the granulation tissue is becoming raised above the wound margin)

3. Evaluate the wound every 2 days to 3 days and apply corticosteroid as needed. Most granulation tissue beds require 1 to 3 applications over a 3-day to 9-day period.

4. Once the granulation tissue has uniformly filled the wound bed and is flush with the skin margin, discontinue application of topical corticosteroid.

5. The skin graft can be performed 4 days to 5 days after the last application of corticosteroid.

treatment of exuberant granulation tissue. Trypsin is a protease enzyme that débrides necrotic tissue; balsam of Peru is a local irritant that is believed to result in improved blood flow; and castor oil may offer some protective effects to the wound bed, promoting epithelialization.[29] Anecdotally, Granulex V (Pfizer Animal Health, New York, NY) has been used to débride exuberant granulation tissue in equine wounds. In December 2015, production of Granulex was discontinued.[34] Alternative products for the aerosol spray include TBC Spray (Delta Pharmaceutical, Irmo, South Carolina), which is a prescription-only product that contains all 3 ingredients present in Granulex, and Proderm (Bertek Pharmaceuticals, Morgantown, WV), which is an over-the-counter aerosol that only contains balsam of Peru and castor oil.[35]

MISCELLANEOUS TOPICAL THERAPIES
Platelet-Rich Plasma Gel

Platelet-rich plasma (PRP) has been used in various medical conditions to improve healing since the late 1980s.[36] Platelets are essential in the initial response to wounding because they promote hemostasis, and, in the later hours to early days of wound healing, they provide growth factors and hydrolytic enzymes (see Linda A. Dahlgren's article, "Regenerative Medicine Therapies for Equine Wound Management", in this issue). Because PRP is made from a patient's own plasma, it is considered safe.[37] One limitation in the use of PRP is the variable presence of white blood cells within the preparation. High white blood cell concentrations in PRP are believed proinflammatory, which could be desirable or detrimental, depending on the phase of wound healing. The development of exuberant granulation tissue on distal limb wounds of horses may result from a retarded inflammatory response. This suggests that the use of leukocyte-rich PRP could have beneficial effects in the treatment of wounds with exuberant granulation tissue. Depletion of leukocytes in PRP preparation, however, does not affect the healing ability of fibroblasts.[38] PRP gel is created by the addition of calcium gluconate plus thrombin to the plasma. The calcium gluconate and thrombin combination can be a platelet activator, thereby mediating growth factor release. When evaluated in experimental models of equine wounds, PRP gel improved epithelial differentiation and collagen organization.[39,40]

Oxygen Therapy

Oxygen is essential to the healing of wounds. Optimization of wound perfusion and oxygenation of tissues are essential for prevention of wound infection. Appropriate oxygen levels, measured by the partial pressure of oxygen surrounding the wound, are essential for normal cellular functions and the ability to generate proper healing responses.[41] Although oxygen is important for wound healing, some level of hypoxia is necessary to promote angiogenesis. The ideal oxygen concentration likely varies with the stage of wound healing and level of damage to the affected tissue. This makes determining correct protocols for topical oxygen therapy difficult. Oxygen delivery via hyperbaric chambers has been used to promote healing for numerous conditions in horses. Hyperbaric chambers allow for the exposure to 100% oxygen in a pressurized environment. Hyperbaric oxygen is used in humans to treat crush injuries, compartment syndrome, diabetic chronic wounds/ulcers, and necrotizing soft tissue infections with varying results.[42] In horses, hyperbaric oxygen therapy is particularly useful in the treatment of clostridial myonecrosis allowing for direct inhibition of the clostridial alpha-toxin and improved microbial killing.[42] Topical oxygen therapy via an electrochemical oxygen concentration device (EPIFLO Transdermal Continuous Oxygen Therapy; Ogenix Corporation, Beachwood, Ohio) has been evaluated in experimental wounds of the distal limbs of horses; however, no difference in wound healing rates or in histologic assessments were noted between the treatment and control groups.[43] Although no differences in wound healing were seen in this study, oxygen therapy could be indicated for some chronic or nonhealing wounds. Ideal application methods and timing of delivery remain to be determined.

Ozone delivery is used to promote oxygenation within the wound bed. Ozone promotes wound healing by increasing fibroblast migration, decreasing inflammation, and up-regulating the production of growth factors.[44] Ozone can inhibit the growth of several common equine wound isolates, such as *E coli*, *S aureus*, and *P aeruginosa*, in culture.[12] Application of topical ozone can occur via 2 methods: (1) by placing the affected region in a sealed, ozone-resistant bag followed by insufflation and (2) by applying ozonized oil directly to the wound (ozone can be stabilized when placed in olive oil).[45] Ozone therapy has not been evaluated in horses. Like oxygen therapy, some equine wounds may benefit from ozone application; however, ideal case selection and timing of administration remain to be determined.

Aloe Vera

Aloe vera is a plant-derived product that is used topically for the treatment of abrasions and wounds. Soothing effects after topical application has been reported in humans. Multiple compounds within the aloe plant provide the benefits seen with its use; however, the main active compound seems to be acemannan. Acemannan stimulates the production of proinflammatory cytokines by macrophages resulting in fibroblast proliferation, epithelialization, and angiogenesis. Numerous human and veterinary products containing acemannan exist, including wound cleansers (EquineVet Acemannan Wound Cleanser, Medline (Carrington Labs, Irving, TX)), sprays, and impregnated gauze dressings. Although no studies have been performed in horses, dog wounds treated with acemannan hydrogels demonstrated improved wound contraction and epithelization.[46]

Scarlet Oil

Scarlet oil is composed of mineral oil, pine oil, eucalyptus oil, isopropyl alcohol 30%, benzyl alcohol 3%, methyl salicylate, parachlorometaxylenol, and scarlet red.[29] Although this compound has been used in the treatment of equine wounds, there is no experimental evidence determining positive or negative effects on wound healing. Scarlet oil is used by veterinarians to hopefully promote the production of granulation tissue, particularly in wounds of the upper body. Some antimicrobial effects may be obtained through the properties of the pine and eucalyptus oils. The use of scarlet oil in horses, however, can result in a substantial contact dermatitis requiring discontinuation of use.[12]

SUMMARY

In conclusion, numerous topical therapies exist for the management of equine wounds. Overall, wounds should be reassessed frequently. The decision of which topical therapies to use should be made based on the stage of wound healing, appearance of the wound, and level of contamination or infection. Combination therapies to enhance healing can be applied where indicated. Topical cleansers and antiseptics are important when treating an acute wound, minimizing bacterial colonization, and with chronic wounds, to prevent infection that can delay wound healing. Topical antimicrobials can be added with or without the addition of a bandage. Continual development of resistant microorganisms demonstrates the importance of minimize systemic antibiotic therapy and controlling local bacterial colonization and infection with topical antimicrobial products, such as honey and octenidine gel. Other topical medications, such as corticosteroids or PRP gels, can be used during specific phases of wound healing to manipulate the wound environment and promote improved and more rapid healing.

REFERENCES

1. Resende MM, Rocha CA, Correa NF, et al. Tap water versus sterile saline solution in the colonisation of skin wounds. Int Wound J 2016;13:526–30.
2. Buffa EA, Lubbe AM, Verstraete FJ, et al. The effects of wound lavage solutions on canine fibroblasts: an in vitro study. Vet Surg 1997;26:460–6.
3. Atiyeh BS, Dibo SA, Hayek SN. Wound cleansing, topical antiseptics and wound healing. Int Wound J 2009;6:420–30.
4. Singer AJ, Hollander JE, Subramanian S, et al. Pressure dynamics of various irrigation techniques commonly used in the emergency department. Ann Emerg Med 1994;24:36–40.
5. Toth T, Brostrom H, Baverud V, et al. Evaluation of LHP(R) (1% hydrogen peroxide) cream versus petrolatum and untreated controls in open wounds in healthy horses: a randomized, blinded control study. Acta Vet Scand 2011;53:45.
6. Angel DE, Morey P, Storer JG, et al. The great debate over iodine in wound care continues: a review fo the literature. Wound Pract Res 2008;16:6–21.
7. Severyns AM, Lejeune A, Rocoux G, et al. Non-toxic antiseptic irrigation with chlorhexidine in experimental revascularization in the rat. J Hosp Infect 1991; 17:197–206.
8. Kramer A, Dissemond J, Kim S, et al. Consensus on wound antisepsis: update 2018. Skin Pharmacol Physiol 2018;31:28–58.
9. Wilson DG, Cooley AJ, MacWilliams PS, et al. Effects of 0.05% chlorhexidine lavage on the tarsocrural joints of horses. Vet Surg 1994;23:442–7.
10. Rani SA, Hoon R, Najafi RR, et al. The in vitro antimicrobial activity of wound and skin cleansers at nontoxic concentrations. Adv Skin Wound Care 2014;27:65–9.
11. Romanowski EG, Stella NA, Yates KA, et al. In vitro evaluation of a hypochlorous acid hygiene solution on established biofilms. Eye Contact Lens 2018. [Epub ahead of print].
12. Jacobsen S. Topical wound treatments and wound-care products. In: Theoret CL, Schumacher J, editors. Equine wound management. 3rd edition. Ames (IA): Wiley-Blackwell; 2017. p. 75–103.
13. Power G, Moore Z, O'Connor T. Measurement of pH, exudate composition and temperature in wound healing: a systematic review. J Wound Care 2017;26:381–97.
14. Wooley RE, Jones MS. Action of EDTA-Tris and antimicrobial agent combinations on selected pathogenic bacteria. Vet Microbiol 1983;8:271–80.
15. Banin E, Brady KM, Greenberg EP. Chelator-induced dispersal and killing of Pseudomonas aeruginosa cells in a biofilm. Appl Environ Microbiol 2006;72: 2064–9.
16. Ashworth CD, Nelson DR. Antimicrobial potentiation of irrigation solutions containing tris-[hydroxymethyl] aminomethane-EDTA. J Am Vet Med Assoc 1990; 197:1513–4.
17. Westgate SJ, Percival SL, Knottenbelt DC, et al. Microbiology of equine wounds and evidence of bacterial biofilms. Vet Microbiol 2011;150:152–9.
18. Peter FW, Li-Peuser H, Vogt PM, et al. The effect of wound ointments on tissue microcirculation and leucocyte behaviour. Clin Exp Dermatol 2002;27:51–5.

19. Bischofberger AS, Tsang AS, Horadagoda N, et al. Effect of activated protein C in second intention healing of equine distal limb wounds: a preliminary study. Aust Vet J 2015;93:361–6.
20. Yabanoglu H, Basaran O, Aydogan C, et al. Assessment of the effectiveness of silver-coated dressing, chlorhexidine acetate (0.5%), citric acid (3%), and silver sulfadiazine (1%) for topical antibacterial effects against the multi-drug resistant Pseudomonas aeruginosa infecting full-skin thickness burn wounds on rats. Int Surg 2013;98:416–23.
21. Berry DB 2nd, Sullins KE. Effects of topical application of antimicrobials and bandaging on healing and granulation tissue formation in wounds of the distal aspect of the limbs in horses. Am J Vet Res 2003;64:88–92.
22. Mavric E, Wittmann S, Barth G, et al. Identification and quantification of methyl-glyoxal as the dominant antibacterial constituent of Manuka (Leptospermum sco-parium) honeys from New Zealand. Mol Nutr Food Res 2008;52:483–9.
23. Tsang AS, Dart AJ, Sole-Guitart A, et al. Comparison of the effects of topical application of UMF20 and UMF5 manuka honey with a generic multifloral honey on wound healing variables in an uncontaminated surgical equine distal limb wound model. Aust Vet J 2017;95:333–7.
24. Bischofberger AS, Dart CM, Perkins NR, et al. The effect of short- and long-term treatment with manuka honey on second intention healing of contaminated and noncontaminated wounds on the distal aspect of the forelimbs in horses. Vet Surg 2013;42:154–60.
25. Carnwath R, Graham EM, Reynolds K, et al. The antimicrobial activity of honey against common equine wound bacterial isolates. Vet J 2014;199:110–4.
26. Fitzgerald DJ, Renick PJ, Forrest EC, et al. Cadexomer iodine provides superior efficacy against bacterial wound biofilms in vitro and in vivo. Wound Repair Re-gen 2017;25:13–24.
27. Ohtani T, Mizuashi M, Ito Y, et al. Cadexomer as well as cadexomer iodine in-duces the production of proinflammatory cytokines and vascular endothelial growth factor by human macrophages. Exp Dermatol 2007;16:318–23.
28. Hammerle G, Strohal R. Efficacy and cost-effectiveness of octenidine wound gel in the treatment of chronic venous leg ulcers in comparison to modern wound dressings. Int Wound J 2016;13:182–8.
29. Farstvedt E, Stashak T, Othic A. Update on topical wound medications. Clin Tech Equine Pract 2004;3:194–272.
30. Hiraku Y, Sekine A, Nabeshi H, et al. Mechanism of carcinogenesis induced by a veterinary antimicrobial drug, nitrofurazone, via oxidative DNA damage and cell proliferation. Cancer Lett 2004;215:141–50.
31. Bello TR. Practical treatment of body and open leg wounds of horses with bovine collagen, biosynthetic wound dressing and cyanoacrylate. J Equine Vet Sci 2002; 22:157–64.
32. Hashimoto I, Nakanishi H, Shono Y, et al. Angiostatic effects of corticosteroid on wound healing of the rabbit ear. J Med Invest 2002;49:61–6.
33. Bailey SR. Corticosteroid-associated laminitis. Vet Clin North Am Equine Pract 2010;26:277–85.
34. Granulex aerosol spray discontinued 2015. Available at: http://www.empr.com/news/granulex-aerosol-spray-discontinued/article/462532/. Accessed April, 2018.
35. Drug discontinuation alert: Granulex® aerosol spray. 2016. Available at: http://files.clickdimensions.com/hospiscriptcom-arzml/files/drugdiscontinuationalerts0104201 6granulexditemp.pdf. Accessed April, 2018.

36. Alves R, Grimalt R. A review of platelet-rich plasma: history, biology, mechanism of action, and classification. Skin Appendage Disord 2018;4:18–24.

37. Lacci KM, Dardik A. Platelet-rich plasma: support for its use in wound healing. Yale J Biol Med 2010;83:1–9.

38. Giusti I, Di Francesco M, D'Ascenzo S, et al. Leukocyte depletion does not affect the in vitro healing ability of platelet rich plasma. Exp Ther Med 2018;15:4029–38.

39. Carter CA, Jolly DG, Worden CE Sr, et al. Platelet-rich plasma gel promotes differentiation and regeneration during equine wound healing. Exp Mol Pathol 2003; 74:244–55.

40. DeRossi R, Coelho AC, Mello GS, et al. Effects of platelet-rich plasma gel on skin healing in surgical wound in horses. Acta Cir Bras 2009;24:276–81.

41. Sen CK. Wound healing essentials: let there be oxygen. Wound Repair Regen 2009;17:1–18.

42. Bhutani S, Vishwanath G. Hyperbaric oxygen and wound healing. Indian J Plast Surg 2012;45:316–24.

43. Tracey AK, Alcott CJ, Schleining JA, et al. The effects of topical oxygen therapy on equine distal limb dermal wound healing. Can Vet J 2014;55:1146–52.

44. Xiao W, Tang H, Wu M, et al. Ozone oil promotes wound healing by increasing the migration of fibroblasts via PI3K/Akt/mTOR signaling pathway. Biosci Rep 2017; 37(6) [pii:BSR20170658].

45. Valacchi G, Fortino V, Bocci V. The dual action of ozone on the skin. Br J Dermatol 2005;153:1096–100.

46. Swaim SF, Riddell KP, Mcguire JA. Effects of topical medications on the healing of open pad wounds in dogs. J Am Anim Hosp Assoc 1992;28:499–502.

Choosing the Best Approach to Wound Management and Closure

Louis Kamus, DMV, MSc[a],*, Christine Theoret, DMV, PhD[b]

KEYWORDS

- Horse • Wound • Primary closure • Secondary intention healing • Delayed closure

KEY POINTS

- Each wound requires an individual assessment to identify the most suitable approach.
- Clear client communication and good knowledge of the healing process are critical to achieving the best possible outcome for the horse.
- Primary closure provides the best cosmetic and functional outcomes for the horse and limits the cost and aftercare required by the owner.
- Second-intention healing is selected to manage wounds with heavy contamination or with extensive trauma/tissue loss.
- Delayed closure can be used when a wound is highly at risk of infection and dehiscence.

INTRODUCTION

Wounds account for a large portion of the caseload of an equine practitioner. The US Department of Agriculture found that skin wounds are the most common medical condition affecting horses[1]; this is also reported by UK horse owners.[2] Similarly, equine veterinarians in New Zealand and Australia report that 25% of their caseload is wound related.[3] In emergency situations, equine ambulatory practitioners often face the dilemma, Should I suture the wound or not? There is no easy answer based on well-defined rules and wound classifications. Each wound must be considered as a unique problem that requires a clinician to take into account all its characteristics to determine the best management approach. The aim of this article is to help the practitioner by providing the tools to decide which type of closure or healing is best in a given situation. An overview of the main criteria and the different approaches to wound closure is presented.

Disclosure Statement: The authors declare no commercial or financial conflicts of interest related to this review.
[a] Clinical Sciences, Faculté de médecine vétérinaire, Université de Montréal, 3200, rue Sicotte, Saint-Hyacinthe, Quebec J2S 2M2, Canada; [b] Faculté de médecine vétérinaire, Université de Montréal, 3200, rue Sicotte, Saint-Hyacinthe, Quebec J2S 2M2, Canada
* Corresponding author.
E-mail address: louis.j.kamus@umontreal.ca

FACTORS THAT INFLUENCE THE CHOICE OF TREATMENT

To select the optimal approach to manage a wound, a full clinical assessment of the patient and a careful examination of the wound are required. The decision to close or not to close a wound should be adapted to each wound and circumstance. Moreover, the veterinarian must recognize that the wound healing process in horses differs from that observed in other mammalian species.[4,5] These differences extend even to ponies, the latter being less susceptible to wound dehiscence, bone sequestrum formation, exuberant granulation tissue (EGT) formation, and delayed wound healing than are horses.[6] Faster and less problematic healing is thus expected for ponies compared with horses. Different factors can influence wound healing and the outcome of treatment; these must be recognized for a clinician to adapt his approach and to anticipate the evolution of the wound. Knowledge of these factors is prerequisite to effective client communication.

Patient-Related Factors

Full consideration of the health of the patient is necessary when attending a wound. Many factors can potentially influence the response to the attempted approach and its outcome. Advanced age of the patient does not seem to directly affect healing in horses.[7] Age-related diseases, however, influencing the systemic state of the patient must be taken into consideration because the consequences could impair healing (eg, Cushing disease). Patients who suffered substantial blood loss or are in shock after trauma may not be good candidates for early treatment of the wound. Rather, stabilization and improvement of the patient's systemic state are often first required to maximize the success of wound management. The nutritional status of the horse is of utmost importance because wound healing is an energy-demanding process. Patients with a negative metabolic status are more likely to experience impeded and failed healing.[7]

Wound-Related Factors

Each wound is unique and should be assessed to select the best approach for treatment. Many practitioners have learned that wounds less than 6 hours to 8 hours old can be closed with low risk of infection and dehiscence. This dogma finds its origin in laboratory animal and human studies from the nineteenth century and from World War II. This golden period concept, however, is no longer considered accurate and each wound must be evaluated in light of several factors in addition to duration.

The choice of treatment of a wound is always related to the wound's location, its type, and degree of compromise to structures underlying the skin. As demonstrated in previous studies comparing horses and ponies, wounds on the distal limb of horses heal differently compared with wounds located on the body.[5] Distal limb wounds usually show a more marked expansion/retraction phase in the early phase of healing,[8] which is followed by inefficient contraction and slow epithelialization.[9] A wound in this location is also more exposed to environmental contamination with foreign material due to its proximity to the ground. Moreover, EGT is more likely to develop in wounds on the distal limb[10] and in areas of high motion. The intrinsic characteristics of the wound (size, depth, orientation, and amount of tissue loss) influence the rate of healing and the selected approach for reconstruction. Similarly, identifying and managing seroma, hematoma, edema, and/or dead space are essential to limit the risk of infection and wound dehiscence. It is of utmost importance to assess the implication of underlying structures during wound evaluation. Wounds with synovial, pleural, abdominal, and/or sinus cavity implications are complicated wounds that may require hospitalization for extensive and aggressive treatment.[7,11] The implication of bone, ligament, or tendon also requires a specific approach; for example, bone exposure and periosteal damage often lead to the formation of a sequestrum during healing (see Randy B. Eggleston's article, "Wound Management: Wounds with Special Challenges," in this issue). The sequestrum acts as a foreign body that impedes healing, promotes inflammation and infection, and encourages the development of EGT.[12] Ligament and tendon are poorly vascularized structures that are, therefore, good foci of uncontrolled infection.[13] Movement of a tendon within a wound promotes formation of different planes of granulation tissue[13] as well as EGT,[12] thereby impeding healing. Wounds involving damage to underlying tendons or ligaments often require immobilization. These particular situations must be recognized to educate owners about their influence on the outcome of the wound management (see Randy B. Eggleston's article, "Equine Wound Management: Bandages, Casts, and External Support," in this issue).

Tissue perfusion around the wound and within the wound bed is critical to an effective healing process. By recognizing situations where blood flow is impeded (eg, trauma to local vessel and hypovolemia), the clinician should adopt an approach to optimize healing and anticipate complications. Optimal tissue perfusion and oxygenation are essential for the elimination of bacteria, collagen synthesis, and epithelialization.[7] Apart from restoring normovolemia when necessary, healing can be optimized by removing avascular and necrotic debris and débriding the wound bed until bleeding healthy tissue is reached.[7] By doing so, healing progresses more quickly and efficiently.[14]

The risk of infection in horses' wounds is high because horses are housed in environments harboring bacterial populations able to colonize open wounds. Moreover, foreign bodies are often found in horses' wounds. Infection is a major cause of dehiscence and delayed wound healing because bacterial enzymes and endotoxins interfere with the healing process and promote chronic inflammation.[7] There is also evidence of the presence of biofilm in equine surgical and accidental chronic wounds, suggesting that biofilm might impair wound healing in horses.[15,16] Early identification of uncontrolled infection, therefore, is critical to avoid the formation of biofilm and delayed healing.[17,18] The quantification of the wound bioburden is often unpractical and unrealistic in many clinical settings and the practitioner must rely on the clinical signs of infection, such as heat, swelling, discharge, odor, and pain from the wounded area. Irregular tissue, reddish tissue, and EGT also can indicate ongoing uncontrolled infection within the wound bed. The first step of effective wound bioburden control involves aggressive débridement, irrigation, proper drainage, and wound protection, when possible (see Karl E. Frees' article, "Equine Practice on Wound Management: Wound Cleansing and Hygiene," and Britta S. Leise's article, "Topical Wound Medications," in this issue). In cases of uncontrolled infection, antimicrobial strategies (antibiotics and specific dressings) combined with wound revisions are recommended (see Britta S. Leise's article, "Topical Wound Medications," and R. Reid Hanson's article, "Medical Therapy in Equine Wound Management," in this issue).

Wounds are frequently managed by owners before a patient is presented to a veterinarian. Knowledge of prior treatments can be helpful to understand and predict the behavior of the wound. Some topical treatments commonly used by horse owners (caustic agents, anti-inflammatory drugs, and antibiotics) may have negative effects on the healing process, depending of the timing and duration of their use.[7]

Taking into account all these factors helps the clinician choose the best approach to wound management and the decision to close or to leave open a defect.

Factors influencing wound management:

- Systemic state
- Concurrent disease
- Nutritional status
- Nature and location of the wound
- Characteristics of the wound
- Involvement of underlying structures
- Tissue perfusion
- Contamination
- Prior treatments

PRIMARY CLOSURE AND DELAYED PRIMARY CLOSURE
Primary Closure

Primary closure refers to closing the wound immediately after cleansing, débriding, establishing proper drainage and immobilization, as needed.[18,19] If successful, this approach provides the best cosmetic and functional outcomes for the horse because bringing wound edges together covers the defect, protects from further contamination, and decreases the amount of tissue repair needed to re-establish skin function and integrity. Primary closure, however, can sometimes fail due to dehiscence caused by infection. A correct wound evaluation and preparation is, therefore, mandatory before any attempt at primary closure.

Scant information is available in the literature regarding the outcome of this type of wound closure in horses. In a retrospective study of first intention healing of traumatic wounds in horses and ponies, more than 60% were located on the distal limb. Primary closure was successful, with no dehiscence, in only 26% of horses and 41% of ponies.[6] Primary closure is also associated with superior cosmetic and positive athletic outcomes in horses with a wound on the distal limb involving traumatic laceration of the extensor tendons.[20] In the authors' personal experience, many wounds treated by primary closure show a minor degree of focal wound dehiscence or infection that can be quickly handled with local therapy. The authors consider these wounds as successfully treated by primary closure.

Primary closure is often the treatment of choice for fresh and minimally contaminated wounds with a good blood supply, moderate tissue loss, and minimal tension on the wound edges.[18] These typically include head, body, and upper limb wounds; wounds with a well-vascularized skin flap; and some distal limb wounds that meet these favorable criteria. Wounds from sharp trauma are also candidates for primary closure. On the other hand, primary closure are not suitable for wounds with the following characteristics: heavy contamination, edema, extensive tissue loss, crush, and abrasive trauma. Nonetheless, some wounds that, in theory, are not good candidates for primary closure because of high contamination or compromised blood supply may still be considered for early suturing. This is usually the case for wounds occurring in the metacarpal/metatarsal area (eg, degloving injury), which suffer from high skin tension and consequently few to no options for reconstruction when allowed to heal by second intention.[21] When primarily closed, the skin flap acts as a temporary biological bandage meant to protect underlying critical structures (bone, tendon, and so forth) from desiccation and to encourage formation of a protective healthy layer of granulation tissue.[18] It is particularly important, in this type of wound, to achieve good control of contamination through débridement and ventral drainage. In these cases, it is critical to prepare the owner for the potential failure and complete dehiscence of the attempted primary closure, a situation ultimately requiring management by either delayed secondary closure (discussed later) or second-intention healing.

Characteristics of wounds suitable for primary closure:

- Minimal contamination
- Good blood supply
- Moderate tissue loss
- Moderate tension on wound edges

Types of wounds:

- Fresh
- Head
- Flap wounds (neck, flank, thorax, and upper limb)
- Sharp trauma
- Some distal limb wounds
- Metacarpal/metatarsal degloving injuries

Tips for successful primary closure:

- Effective débridement and irrigation
- Reduction of dead space
- Proper drainage
- Relief of tension
- Minimization of suture material
- Immobilization, when possible

Delayed Primary Closure

In many situations, as an alternative to first-intention healing, closure can be delayed for a few days (1–3 days) to allow better preparation of the wound bed to increase the chance of success of closure. This is referred to as delayed primary closure.[18] Repeated débridement and irrigation reduce the bacterial burden and prevent the formation of biofilm.[17] Specific types of dressing material and antimicrobial therapies also can be used during this period of delay, to manage infection (see Britta S. Leise's article, "Topical Wound Medications," and R. Reid Hanson's article, "Medical Therapy in Equine Wound Management," in this issue). Edema can be managed with hypertonic saline dressings.

To the authors' knowledge, no studies have been conducted in horses to assess if a superior outcome can be expected after delayed primary closure compared with primary closure. The medical literature suggests that delayed primary closure may reduce the occurrence of surgical site infection in specific wound scenarios in human patients, but definitive evidence has yet to be provided.[22–24] A recent systematic review from the Cochrane database concluded that there is currently no evidence to guide clinical decision making regarding the timing for closure of traumatic wounds.[25] Repeated débridement and irrigation prior to closure, however, are certainly beneficial because wounds in horses are subject to heavy contamination.[7]

The major drawback of delayed primary closure is that the veterinarian must deal with the initial wound expansion that occurs in the first weeks of healing in horses.[5] This gradual increase in size of the wound surface area could impede complete closure of the wound but, ultimately, partial closure still is preferable to second-intention healing. It may be possible, in some cases, to limit wound expansion by placing retention sutures across the wound gap during the waiting period or by undermining a wound's edges before undertaking delayed primary closure.[18]

Delayed primary closure is a suitable approach for wounds that could be closed by primary closure but are heavily contaminated or excessively swollen, thereby increasing the likelihood of dehiscence. This is the case, for example, of limb wounds with extensive soft tissue trauma and inflammation due to struggling[18] or of wounds located over open synovial cavities (see Elsa K. Ludwig and Philip D. van Harreveld's article, "Equine Wounds Over Synovial Structures," in this issue). Delayed primary closure could also be indicated for patients who suffered substantial blood loss or are in shock after the trauma. When a patient's systemic state improves and stabilizes, wound closure can be safely attempted.

Characteristics of wounds suitable for delayed primary closure:

- Up to 1 day to 3 days after trauma
- Wounds suitable for primary closure but with marked
  - Contamination
  - Edema
  - Drainage
- Substantial blood loss
- Shock

Tips for successful delayed primary closure:

- Repeated débridement and irrigation
- Use of hypertonic saline dressings
- Use of antimicrobial therapies
- Use of retention sutures
- Tissue undermining

SECOND-INTENTION HEALING AND DELAYED SECONDARY CLOSURE
Second-Intention Healing

In most cases when primary or delayed primary closures are not an option, it is because the wound is grossly contaminated and/or suffering moderate to severe tissue loss. Apposition of the wound edges, therefore, is not possible and wounds must heal through granulation, contraction, and epithelialization. This type of healing is referred to as second-intention healing.[18] Second-intention healing also pertains to wounds that have undergone partial or complete dehiscence of a primary closure. These wounds still require good débridement and cleansing to reduce contamination or infection as well as proper ventral drainage. Second-intention management often requires multiple interventions to stimulate and control the progression of healing, because they are more prone to prolonged healing time. Immobilization, when possible, may be necessary to minimize damage to the wound bed caused by motion (see Randy B. Eggleston's article, "Equine Wound Management: Bandages, Casts, and External Support," in this issue). This wound management approach might be chosen by owners concerned by the cost of an initial primary or delayed primary closure. Costs associated with multiple and repeated veterinary interventions required to ensure proper healing, however, may surpass those of a successful primary closure.

Second-intention healing is not ideal because wounds in horses heal primarily by epithelialization rather than by wound contraction, especially when located on the limb.[9] This leads to the formation of a more extensive and weaker scar (that can withstand a maximum load of only 60% of the breaking force of normal intact skin[26]), in which normal skin adnexa (pigmentation, hair, sweat, and sebaceous glands) are not regenerated.[8] Body wounds usually heal with an acceptable functional and cosmetic outcome, except for those involving severe trauma with extensive tissue loss.[18] Body wounds also heal significantly faster than do wounds on the limbs.[9] Wounds on the distal aspect of the limb heal poorly by second intention and often form EGT,[6] which require multiple débridements to allow epithelialization and contraction to ensue.

Wounds with extensive tissue loss and gross contamination require second-intention management.[18] This also is normally the approach selected for wounds of the axilla and groin as well as burn injuries and wounds caused by pressure or entrapment.[18] Degloving injuries of the limb, which suffer partial or complete dehiscence after primary closure, must also heal by second intention.[21]

Characteristics of wounds suitable for second-intention healing:

- Gross contamination
- Extensive tissue loss
- High tension on wound edges

Specific types of wounds:

- Axilla
- Groin
- Burn injuries
- Pressure/entrapment injuries
- Metacarpal/metatarsal degloving injuries

Tips for second-intention healing:

- Effective débridement and irrigation
- Proper drainage
- Immobilization, when possible
- Early stimulation of fibroplasia/granulation
- Trimming of EGT

Delayed Secondary Closure

Once a bed of healthy granulation tissue has filled a wound defect when healing by second intention, it is possible to attempt to bring together and suture the wound edges. This is referred to as delayed secondary closure.[18] The goal is to speed up the healing process, to avoid the formation (or recurrence) of EGT, and to aim for a more cosmetic and functional outcome. Delayed secondary closure requires a combination of partial resection of granulation tissue, undermining of wound edges, tension-relieving suture patterns, proper distal drainage, and, in some cases, immobilization of the treated area. Delayed secondary closure is suitable for wounds having a limited loss of tissue and presenting healthy granulation tissue (absence of infection, smooth, and well vascularized).

Delayed secondary closure is often chosen for heavily contaminated or infected wounds that have previously been managed by an owner. Common examples are heel bulb or pastern lacerations.[18,27] These types of wounds heal well with delayed secondary closure supported by proper immobilization (cast) (see Randy B. Eggleston's article, "Wound Management: Bandages, Casts, and External Support," in this issue). Delayed secondary closure can also be used for revision of chronic wounds. Delayed secondary closure is not, however, suitable for wounds in areas of high skin tension (eg, metacarpal/metatarsal area) or characterized by severe loss of tissue.[18]

Characteristics of wounds suitable for delayed secondary closure:

- Revision of wounds healing by second intention
- Healthy granulation tissue
- Minimal skin tension

Tips for successful delayed primary closure:

- Trimming of granulation tissue
- Proper drainage
- Undermining
- Tension-relieving suture patterns
- Immobilization

SUMMARY

Unfortunately, there is no simple and straightforward algorithm (**Fig. 1**) to determine if a wound should be closed or not. Each wound requires an individual assessment to identify the most suitable approach. Many factors determine the rate and outcome of the

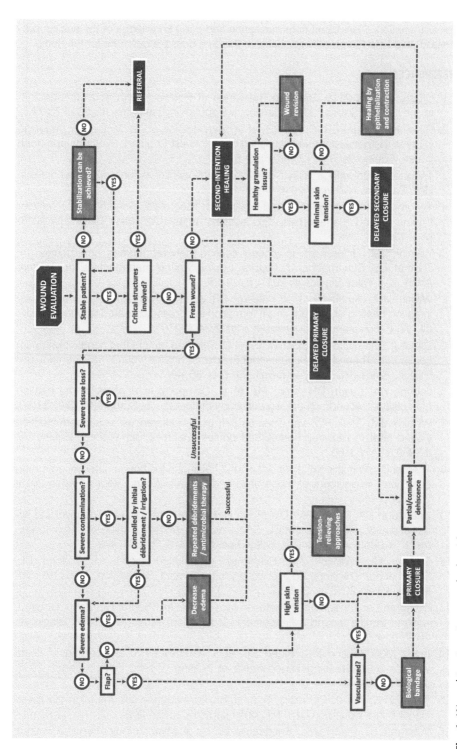

Fig. 1. Wound treatment approach algorithm.

healing process and these must be identified when a wounded horse is first presented for examination. Clear client communication and good knowledge of the healing process should help the practitioner achieve the best possible outcome for the horse.

REFERENCES

1. USDA. Equine 2015: Baseline Reference of Equine Health and Management in the United States, 2015. Section I: Population Estimates In: 2015:73-77.
2. Owen KR, Singer ER, Clegg PD, et al. Identification of risk factors for traumatic injury in the general horse population of north-west England, Midlands and north Wales. Equine Vet J 2012;44(2):143-8.
3. Theoret CL, Bolwell CF, Riley CB. A cross-sectional survey on wounds in horses in New Zealand. N Z Vet J 2016;64:90-4.
4. Theoret CL. Physiology of wound healing. In: Theoret CL, Schumacher J, editors. Equine wound management. 3rd edition. Ames (IA): Wiley Blackwell; 2017. p. 1-13.
5. Wilmink JM. Differences in wound healing between horses and ponies. In: Theoret CL, Schumacher J, editors. Equine wound management. 3rd editon. Ames (IA): Wiley Blackwell; 2017. p. 14-29.
6. Wilmink JM, van Herten J, van Weeren PR, et al. Retrospective study of primary intention healing and sequestrum formation in horses compared to ponies under clinical circumstances. Equine Vet J 2002;34(3):270-3.
7. Dart AJ, Sole-Guitart A, Stashak TS, et al. Selected factors that negatively impact healing. In: Theoret CL, Schumacher J, editors. Equine wound management. 3rd edition. Ames (IA): Wiley Blacwell; 2017. p. 30-46.
8. Jacobs KA, Leach DH, Fretz PB, et al. Comparative aspects of the healing of excisional wounds on the leg and body of horses. Vet Surg 1984;13(2):83-90.
9. Wilmink JM, Stolk PW, van Weeren PR, et al. Differences in second-intention wound healing between horses and ponies: macroscopic aspects. Equine Vet J 1999;31(1):53-60.
10. Theoret CL, Wilmink JM. Aberrant wound healing in the horse: naturally occurring conditions reminiscent of those observed in man. Wound Repair Regen 2013; 21(3):365-71.
11. Seabaugh KA, Baxter GM. Diagnosis and management of wounds involving synovial structures. In: Theoret CL, Schumacher J, editors. Equine wound management. 3rd edition. Ames (IA): Wiley Blackwell; 2017. p. 385-402.
12. Theoret CL, Wilmink JM. Exuberant granulation tissue. In: Theoret CL, Schumacher J, editors. Equine wound management. 3rd edition. Ames (IA): Wiley Blackwell; 2017. p. 369-84.
13. Dahlgren LA. Tendon and paratenon lacerations. In: Theoret CL, Schumacher J, editors. Equine wound management. 3rd edition. Ames (IA): Wiley Blackwell; 2017. p. 403-21.
14. Franz MG, Robson MC, Steed DL, et al. Guidelines to aid healing of acute wounds by decreasing impediments of healing. Wound Repair Regen 2008; 16(6):723-48.
15. Freeman K, Woods E, Welsby S, et al. Biofilm evidence and the microbial diversity of horse wounds. Can J Microbiol 2009;55(2):197-202.
16. Westgate SJ, Percival SL, Knottenbelt DC, et al. Microbiology of equine wounds and evidence of bacterial biofilms. Vet Microbiol 2011;150(1-2):152-9.

17. Dart AJ, Sole-Guitart A, Stashak TS, et al. Management practices that influence wound infection and healing. In: Theoret CL, Schumacher J, editors. Equine wound management. 3rd edition. Ames (IA): Wiley Blackwell; 2017. p. 47–74.
18. Elce YA. Approaches to wound closure. In: Theoret CL, Schumacher J, editors. Equine wound management. 3rd edition. Ames (IA): Wiley Blackwell; 2017. p. 157–72.
19. Celeste C. Selection of suture materials, suture patterns, and drains for wound closure. In: Theoret CL, Schumacher J, editors. Equine wound management. 3rd edition. Ames (IA): Wiley Blackwell; 2017. p. 173–99.
20. Mespoulhes-Riviere C, Martens A, Bogaert L, et al. Factors affecting outcome of extensor tendon lacerations in the distal limb of horses. A retrospective study of 156 cases (1994-2003). Vet Comp Orthop Traumatol 2008;21(4):358–64.
21. Hanson RR, Schumacher J. Degloving injuries of the distal aspect of the limb. In: Theoret CL, Schumacher J, editors. Equine wound management. 3rd edition. Ames (IA): Wiley Blackwell; 2017. p. 352–68.
22. Bhangu A, Singh P, Lundy J, et al. Systemic review and meta-analysis of randomized clinical trials comparing primary vs delayed primary skin closure in contaminated and dirty abdominal incisions. JAMA Surg 2013;148(8):779–86.
23. Siribumrungwong B, Noorit P, Wilasrusmee C, et al. A systematic review and meta-analysis of randomised controlled trials of delayed primary wound closure in contaminated abdominal wounds. World J Emerg Surg 2014;9(1):49.
24. Siribumrungwong B, Srikuea K, Thakkinstian A. Comparison of superficial surgical site infection between delayed primary and primary wound closures in ruptured appendicitis. Asian J Surg 2014;37(3):120–4.
25. Eliya-Masamba MC, Banda GW. Primary closure versus delayed closure for non bite traumatic wounds within 24 hours post injury. Cochrane Database Syst Rev 2013;(10):CD008574.
26. Monteiro SO, Lepage OM, Theoret CL. Effects of platelet-rich plasma on the repair of wounds on the distal aspect of the forelimb in horses. Am J Vet Res 2009;70(2):277–82.
27. Schumacher J, Stashak TS. Management of wounds of the distal extremities. In: Theoret CL, Schumacher J, editors. Equine wound management. 3rd edition. Ames (IA): Wiley Blackwell; 2017. p. 312–51.

Wound Management
Wounds with Special Challenges

Randy B. Eggleston, DVM

KEYWORDS

- Wound • Musculoskeletal • Genital

KEY POINTS

- Distal limb wounds in horses heal substantially different than trunk wounds, commonly resulting in exuberant granulation tissue and exposed and sequestered bone.
- Surgical intervention of severe rectovaginal lacerations in the mare should be delayed until the tissues have heeled and scar tissue has remodeled.
- Wounds resulting in severe hemorrhage require appropriate emergent fluid therapy and potentially transfusion therapy.

INTRODUCTION

Wound healing in horses typically follows all of the principles of wound healing with a few exceptions. Because of horses' size, environment, and fight-or-flight response to noxious stimuli, wounds commonly involve considerable tissue damage and loss, and high-impact trauma.

Several factors contribute to the challenges of wound management, including the location, size, and depth of the wound, presence of severe hemorrhage, and what underlying tissues are involved in the wound.[1] It is imperative that the veterinarian possesses a strong working knowledge of anatomy and wound healing. These factors can have a substantial impact on how the wound should be managed in the acute stages both diagnostically and therapeutically. They can also give rise to long-term complications if appropriate management was not performed in the early stages. The equine practitioner is commonly confronted with wounds that present unique challenges either at the time of wounding or as the healing process progresses. This article addresses complications commonly associated with the following types of wounds: (1) degloving wounds resulting in exposed bone, (2) wounds with severe hemorrhage, (3) wounds located over areas of high motion, and (4) wounds of the genitalia.

The author has nothing to disclose.
Department of Large Animal Medicine, College of Veterinary Medicine, University of Georgia, 2200 College Station Road, Athens, GA 30602, USA
E-mail address: egglesto@uga.edu

Vet Clin Equine 34 (2018) 511–538
https://doi.org/10.1016/j.cveq.2018.07.003
0749-0739/18/© 2018 Elsevier Inc. All rights reserved.

DISTAL LIMB: DEGLOVING WOUNDS

The location of a wound can have major consequences to the successful management and overall quality of healing. Wounds located over the trunk rarely give rise to management complications because of the amount of underlying soft tissue and the ability of the healing tissues to contract and heal with little scar formation, depending on the overall size of the wound. Wounds to the trunk become complicated when they are located over the dorsum, result in marked tissue loss, or enter the thoracic or peritoneal cavities (**Fig. 1**). Wounds to the head can result in similar complications as those on the distal limb in that tissue manipulation, wound contraction, and epithelialization can be limited. Location of a wound can also make it difficult to take advantage of bandaging with respect to debridement, environment control, and protection.

The distal limb is a very common site of injury in the horse,[2] and injury here can result in some of the more complicated wounds that the equine practitioner can face. Complications in management arise from the lack of overlying soft tissue, which commonly results in involvement of bone, tendon, ligament, neurovascular tissues, and synovial cavities (**Fig. 2**). There are also marked differences in the healing properties of distal limb wounds compared with wounds located over the rest of the body.[3–6]

Notable differences exist in the rate and quality of wound healing between horses and ponies. Immediately after wounding, wound retraction in horses is prolonged and results in a much larger wound, whereas in ponies retraction is limited and results in minimal wound enlargement. The inflammatory phase in ponies is rapid, strong, and efficient, whereas in horses, is weak and persists as chronic inflammation. This in turn results in healthier granulation tissue formation, more efficient and organized fibroblast differentiation, and improved wound contraction in ponies, and persistent fibroplasia, poor wound contraction, and exuberant granulation tissue (EGT) formation in horses. Because of this delayed, disorganized, and inefficient process, the requirement for epithelialization in horses is greater, resulting in a thin, poor-quality epithelium and greater scar formation.[7,8]

Wound Assessment

An in-depth description of wound assessment is included in Earl M. Gaughan's article, "Diagnostic Approaches to Understanding Equine Limb Wounds," and Karl E. Frees's article, "Equine Practice on Wound Management Wound Cleansing and Hygiene," in this issue of this text.

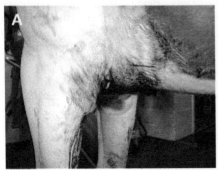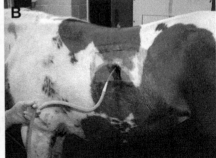

Fig. 1. (*A*) Small axillary wound created by a T-post. Injury entered thoracic cavity resulting in pneumothorax. (*B*) Chest tube placed in left hemithorax for evacuation of pneumothorax.

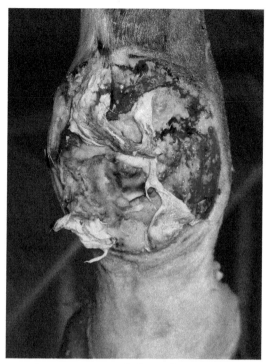

Fig. 2. Distal limb wound over metacarpophalangeal joint. Wound involves the common digital extensor tendon, distal metacarpus, proximal first phalanx, and metacarpophalangeal joint.

Imaging can aid in identifying synovial involvement but can be misleading. Radiography can identify intra-articular gas; however, gas within the overlying affected tissues can sometimes be misinterpreted as intra-articular gas. Placing a metallic probe into the depths of the wound can help evaluate the depth and direction of a wound and proximity to surrounding synovial structures, but it is also not very sensitive in definitively identifying communication. Ultrasound can be useful in identifying joint sepsis and disruption of a synovial tissue but is not always definitive in its findings.[9,10]

Common techniques that can help definitively identify synovial communication include positive contrast radiography (arthrogram, fistulogram) or direct infusion of sterile fluid into the suspected cavity to identify cavity leakage. There is risk in performing these techniques in many cases because of severe tissue damage and cellulitis surrounding the cavity to be investigated. The risk of introducing microorganisms into an otherwise sterile environment is possible with the arthrogram and infusion techniques; with the fistulogram, the risk is with a false negative result when in actuality the synovial cavity has been violated. (See Elsa K. Ludwig and Philip D. van Harreveld's article, "Equine Wounds over Synovial Structures," in this issue.)

Exuberant Granulation Tissue

The major differences in distal limb wound healing include greater post-wounding retraction, persistent chronic inflammation, formation of EGT, and increased epithelialization. In the early inflammatory and debridement phase of healing, distal limb wounds can almost double their original size.[11,12] As healing progresses and a wound defect fills with granulation tissue and the wound contracts completely, fibroplasia ceases. In distal limb wounds, due in part to a weak initial and persistent chronic inflammatory phase, normal fibroblast differentiation is delayed, inefficient, and disorganized, resulting in delayed contraction. The delay in wound contraction and exposed granulation tissue causes persistent chronic inflammation and expression of transforming growth factor-ß1, which further delays wound healing by favoring the formation of EGT and delayed epithelialization.[3–5,8] (See K. Leann Kuebelbeck and Michael Maher's article, "Non-healing Wounds of the Equine Limb," in this issue.)

Bone Sequestration

Degloving wounds commonly extend to the bony structures and usually include some degree of denuded bone or stripping of the periosteal covering.

Once the blood supply to the underlying bone is disrupted, the affected bone becomes ischemic and eventually dies. The devitalized bone becomes sequestered and a nidus for inflammation and infection. Desiccation of the bone also contributes to the sequestration of bone. As long as the sequestered bone is present, normal healing will not progress to cover the affected area[13–16] (**Fig. 3**). Fibroplasia will continue, and granulation tissue forms from the margins of the wound. Future sequestrum formation is not always obvious with visual inspection. Depending on wound location, granulation tissue may cover the bone. A lack of underlying supportive, viable tissue in the distal limb often dictates an incomplete filling of the wound site with granulation tissue. Granulation tissue in these situations often lacks adhesion to the underlying bone, and a linear defect in the granulation bed forms over the sequestered bone. The sequestrum, acting as a foreign body, can become walled off from parent bone forming an involucrum.[16] The initial evidence that a sequestrum is present is persistent inflammation and local infection, resulting in a draining nonhealing wound. Wounds sutured over a sequestrum often become swollen and eventually dehisce and drain. Sequestra commonly do not cause lameness. Depending on the size of the sequestered bone, resorption of the affected bone can occur over a prolonged period of time. If a sequestrum is not confined within an involucrum, the sequestered bone may also be expelled from the wound (**Fig. 4**). In the author's opinion, this does not occur often. Because of persistent inflammation and debris surrounding the affected

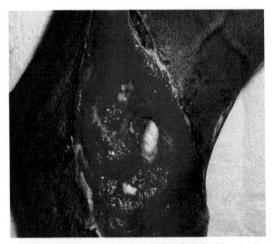

Fig. 3. Chronic granulating degloving wound of the distal tibia. Desiccated discolored sequestrum in the center of the wound is preventing complete granulation tissue coverage and delayed healing.

bone, and an inadequate blood supply preventing an adequate immune response, the time required for natural resolution of the lesion is prolonged and can lead to additional complications with the overall healing of the wound.[15] Most cases require surgical removal of the sequestrum for the wound to heal appropriately.

Depending on the cause of the wound, and the force involved, radiographic assessment may be indicated to more thoroughly evaluate bony structures for possible non-displaced fractures. Radiographs are also indicated for identification of sequestra

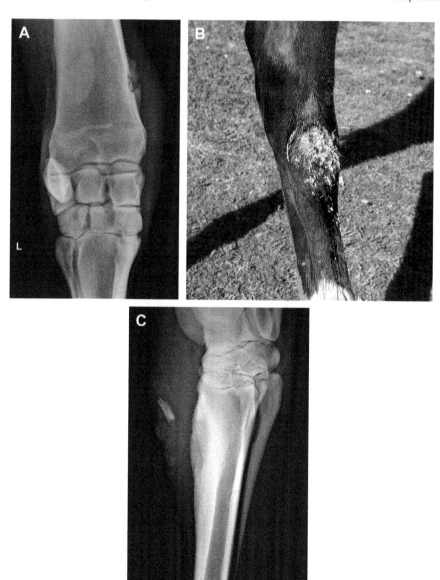

Fig. 4. (*A*) Horse with a chronic nonhealing draining wound to the left front distal medial radius. Well-organized bone sequestrum encased in involucrum. (*B*) Horse with a chronic nonhealing wound to the left hind proximal dorsal metatarsus. (*C*) Radiograph of horse in (*B*) showing bone sequestrum being expelled from wound.

formation. However, radiographs taken within the initial 14 to 21 days after wounding may be unremarkable because of inadequate lysis surrounding the sequestrum. As devitalized bone undergoes necrosis, it becomes detached from the parent bone and can become radiographically apparent as a mineral opacity surrounded by soft tissue opacity.[14,15,17] Proper alignment of radiographic projections is important; aligning the beam angle perpendicular to the wound or the draining tract is optimal for accurate identification of a sequestrum. Depending on the maturity of the bone lesion, small sequestra can be difficult to see if the appropriate radiographic projection is not made.

The decision for wound closure is often influenced by the potential for bone sequestration. The degree of periosteal involvement is fairly obvious at the time of examination, but the potential for osseous sequestration is not always obvious. If denuded bone is present, the wound is clean, and there are no obvious cortical defects, primary closure may be acceptable. Closed skin can act as a biologic bandage, preventing further gross contamination and desiccation of the wound. If affected bone is nonviable and a sequestrum forms, swelling and drainage will occur and a sutured wound will likely dehisce. If this happens, the sequestrum should be removed, and the wound should be left to heal by second intention.

Sequestrectomy is straightforward and can often be completed with a horse standing. If the sequestrum is chronic, there is a tendency for the involucrum to proliferate and form a cloaca that is smaller that the sequestrum, thus entrapping the sequestered bone. In this case, performing the sequestrectomy under general anesthesia should be considered.

Removal of a sequestrum involves identifying its location and configuration. Radiographs can determine sequestra dimensions. Examination of the wound will usually reveal a defect in an incomplete granulation bed. Probing the granulation tissue defect will lead to the area of sequestered bone. Redundant granulation tissue can be removed, and overlying granulation tissue is usually not adhered to the sequestered bone. The sequestered bone is usually discolored and can be loose. Removing more of the granulation tissue will reveal a clear demarcation between the margin of necrotic and healthy bone. A periosteal elevator or bone curette can elevate the sequestrum for removal.[13]

Treatment

Once a wound is completely evaluated, decisions for the most appropriate treatment can be made. A large portion of a treatment plan is going to be based on wound chronicity, involvement of any vital anatomy, size and location of the wound, and the stability of the patient.

Most degloving wounds are the result of substantial trauma and associated with marked tissue damage and contamination. Debridement is the stage of treatment whereby a veterinarian has the greatest impact on the overall management and healing of a wound. Wound debridement involves removal of foreign and organic material, necrotic tissue, and microbial contamination. Debridement methods include lavage, surgical, chemical, and use of bandages. Mechanical debridement is most common during the initial stages of treatment. Following initial debridement, lavage and bandage debridement can be used. Wound lavage should be performed with sterile balanced electrolyte solutions, such as lactated Ringers solution or sodium chloride. Adding a small quantity of antiseptic solution to the lavage solution is commonly done. The lavage solution should be applied under moderate pressure ($\sim$8 psi) at an oblique angle. Using a 19-gauge needle attached to a 35-mL syringe will deliver $\sim$8 psi of pressure (**Fig. 5**). Detergents and alcohol should be avoided in open wounds, because they are detrimental to exposed, viable tissues.[18,19] Dilute povidone iodine and

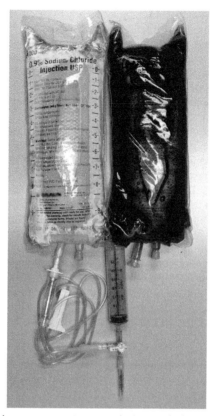

Fig. 5. Wound cleaning lavage system. Lavage solutions include a 0.025% chlorhexidine and a 0.01% betadine solution. Delivery system includes a drip set attached the side port of a 3-way stopcock. A 35-mL syringe and an 18-gauge hypodermic needle are attached to opposing ports. This system is a closed system and allows for multiple cleanings.

chlorhexidine diacetate, delivered under pressure (14 psi), have also been shown to significantly reduce the bacterial load on bone when compared with saline alone.[18] The needed volume of lavage solution will be dictated by the degree of contamination and debris within the wound and wound size. Mechanical debridement may be required over several days as wounded tissue viability is determined.[19,20] (See Karl E. Frees's article, "Equine Practice on Wound Management Wound Cleansing and Hygiene," in this issue.)

If a wound is clean following debridement, primary closure should be considered. Large wounds of the trunk are more conducive to primary closure than those in the distal limb. Larger flap wounds of the distal limb often require tension-relieving and skin mobilization techniques (ie, releasing incisions) to obtain complete closure.[21,22] (See Louis Kamus and Christine Theoret's article, "Choosing the Best Approach to Wound Management and Closure," in this issue.) If substantial tissue loss occurs at the time of wounding, or the result of aggressive wound debridement prevents the possibility of primary closure, second intention management should be considered.

Second intention healing of the equine distal limb often results in EGT. Multiple treatments have been evaluated for management of EGT with minimal positive results.[23–27] Covering distal limb wounds that are healing by second intention promotes an environment conducive to the formation of EGT.[5,24,27–29] Experimentally controlled wounds that are left unbandaged form far less if any EGT, but do result in slightly more scarring, and delay in healing, than bandaged wounds.[27,30] Interestingly, studies comparing bandaged and unbandaged wounds whereby the EGT was excised as needed showed no difference in the overall healing time.[27] When the quality of wound healing is taken into consideration, the added benefits of reduced contamination, trauma, and desiccation that bandages offer surpass the benefits of leaving a wound unbandaged. (See K. Leann Kuebelbeck and Michael Maher's article, "Non-healing Wounds of the Equine Limb," in this issue.)

For wounds that are located over areas of excessive movement (wounds over joints, heel bulb wounds), immobilization of that portion of the limb with a cast or cast bandage can help to significantly reduce the formation of EGT and the number of times that EGT must be excised. (See Randy B. Eggleston's article, "Equine Wound Management: Bandages, Casts, and External Support," in this issue.)

Silicone dressings are used extensively in human medicine in burn patients and for the prevention and treatment of hypertrophic scars and keloids.[31–33] Silicone sheet dressings can be useful in controlling the formation of EGT in horses.[23,34,35]

Topical corticosteroids can also reduce the formation of EGT.[36] However, steroids have an overall negative effect on wound healing by reducing angiogenesis, contraction, and epithelialization.[36–38] Therefore, it is recommended that steroids be used judiciously early in the formation of granulation tissue and use be limited to 1 or 2 applications.[39]

Excision of the protruding granulation tissue is the mainstay of controlling EGT. Excision of EGT is usually required every 3 to 5 days. Excising the proliferative tissue is straightforward and is most commonly done with a horse standing. A no. 20 scalpel blade works well. EGT does not require local anesthesia because of the lack of nervous tissue in granulation tissue. The line of excision should be approximately 2 mm inside the new visible epithelium. A disposable razor can also be used for small-volume EGT excision (**Fig. 6**). The plastic guard distal to the cutting edge can be removed; otherwise, tissue removal is slow and less productive. Marked bleeding will occur during the shaving process. After debridement, the wound should be bandaged with a sterile, nonadherent dressing as the primary layer and an overlying padded pressure bandage. The volume of hemorrhage from debridement usually dictates the bandage be changed the following day.

Chronic wounds that fail to respond to the appropriate treatment or appear to have changed in appearance may be better understood with biopsy of the apparent EGT. Although uncommon, some chronic wounds have developed neoplastic tissue, sarcoid being the most common. If presented with chronic proliferative tissue at a wound site, sarcoid, squamous cell carcinoma, and cutaneous habronemiasis should be ruled in or out as potential causes of a chronic nonhealing wound[40,41] (**Fig. 7**).

WOUNDS RESULTING IN MARKED HEMORRHAGE

Acute blood loss is common with equine wounds and especially after laceration to major arteries and veins. Marked loss can happen after massive tissue trauma to major muscle groups of the trunk or wounds associated with high-velocity trauma, such as collisions with motor vehicles or major falls. Hemothorax or hemoabdomen can result (**Fig. 8**). Fortunately, blood loss from the most equine wounds does not warrant aggressive replacement therapy. The most common site for vascular trauma in the distal limb is laceration of the palmar/plantar digital vessels. Other sites of potential vascular trauma include the lateral metatarsus (greater metatarsal artery), the medial aspect of the radius (cephalic vein), and the medial aspect of the tarsus (saphenous vein).

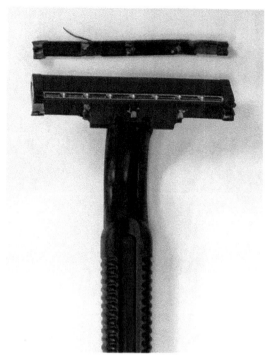

Fig. 6. Disposable razors work well for debridement of EGT. Removal of the plastic guard distal to the blades allows for more affective tissue removal.

Evaluation after vascular trauma should involve a quick assessment of the horse's wound and the site of the trauma. If there is active hemorrhage occurring, it should be addressed first. Evaluating the wound site can give some idea of blood loss, although an accurate prediction of volume is difficult. If there is active bleeding, attempts should be made to identify the responsible vessel and apply clamps and ligatures. Locating the vessel is often difficult due to retraction of the vessel into the soft tissue after transection. If the vessel cannot be located, placing a well-padded pressure bandage can slow and often stop the bleeding. Plenty of time for clotting to occur should be allowed before removing the bandage because removing it too soon will often disrupt the clot and result in continued bleeding. If substantial blood loss occurs with pressure therapy, exploration of the wound under general anesthesia may be indicated. Bandages should be maintained during anesthesia induction to minimize additional rapid blood loss. A thorough physical examination should be performed before general anesthesia to assess the systemic status of the horse to help guide additional supportive therapy deemed necessary while under anesthesia.[14,15,42] A tourniquet placed proximal to the wound is also a very effective hemostatic method.[43] Establishing hemostasis to injured vessels over the trunk is accomplished through direct pressure, or the depth of the wound may allow for packing of the defect and compression of the affected vessels. Severe hemorrhage from abdominal wounds can often be controlled with a tight abdominal bandage. Proximal axial wounds to the limbs and deep wounds to the ventral neck involving the major vasculature are often fatal because of the size of affected vasculature and difficulty in establishing adequate hemostasis in a timely fashion.[44]

Once the bleeding is controlled and blood loss is considered substantial, the horse should be reevaluated for signs of hypovolemic shock. Acute hemorrhage can be

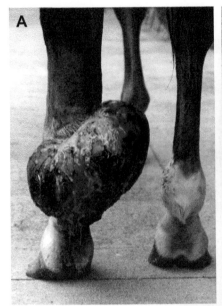
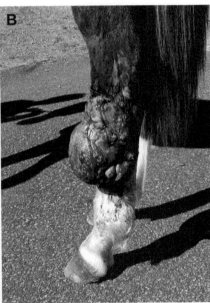
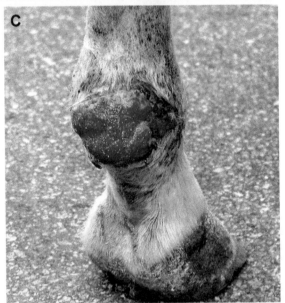

Fig. 7. (A) Three similar-appearing proliferative wounds on the distal limbs of horses. Histologic examination revealed 3 different lesions: (A) EGT, (B) pythiosis (*Pythium insidiosum*), and (C) sarcoid.

internal or external. Internal hemorrhage can be difficult to fully appreciate because of the lack of visible blood loss. The true systemic affects of marked hemorrhage may not present for 12 to 24 hours following the trauma.[43,45]

Clinical signs of hemorrhagic shock will vary depending on the degree of blood loss. With low-volume blood loss (<15% of blood volume), stable compensation is likely provided hemostasis has been established and there are no ongoing losses.[45,46]

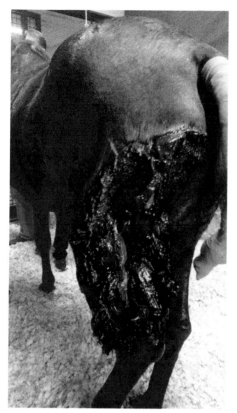

Fig. 8. Mare sustained severe trauma and blood loss after being struck by a pickup truck. Significant portion of the biceps femoris, semimembranosus, and the entire semitendinosus were lacerated. The common perineal (fibular) nerve was also transected.

Volume deficits can be reestablished with little change in the horse's overall physical examination parameters. There may be a normal to slight increase in capillary refill time (CRT), heart rate, and respiratory rate. The horse's hematocrit and total solids may also be normal, and a slight increase in blood lactate can occur. With moderate blood loss (15%–30% of blood volume), clinical signs consistent with hypovolemic shock can be present, including moderate tachycardia and tachypnea, prolonged CRT, bounding pulses, and cool extremities. An affected horse may also show signs of agitation, anxiety, and sweating. It is important to accurately recognize these signs and address them early because compensatory mechanisms may not be able to reestablish normal blood pressure, and perfusion deficits will most likely persist. In cases of severe blood loss (>30%, decompensatory shock), clinical signs will be pronounced. Pulse pressure will be weak along with a severely prolonged CRT and poor jugular refill. Despite increases in heart rate, cardiac contractility, and peripheral resistance, the blood pressure will decrease and remain low because of a lack of compensatory capabilities.[43,45,46] Horses with voluminous hemoperitoneum may also show signs of colic and abdominal distention.[43,46]

Once hemostasis is established, a decision must be made on emergency resuscitation. This decision will be based on the clinical evaluation of the patient (tachycardia, tachypnea, pale mucous membranes, prolonged CRT, and mentation). Hematological indices may also be used to help determine the hydration status and the severity of anemia. However, packed cell volume (PCV) and total protein may be within the normal range for the first 8 to 12 hours following injury while fluid redistribution is occurring.[43,46]

Treatment

Fluid resuscitation

The goals of treating hypovolemic shock due to acute blood loss include the following:

- Establish hemostasis
- Improve cardiac output
- Improve oxygen caring capacity

Fluid therapy is critical to the latter 2 goals. Of the 2, improving cardiac output takes priority over correcting anemia.[46,47] Improved cardiac output increases vascular volume and tissue perfusion.

Isotonic crystalloid fluids (Normosol R, Plasma-Lyte A, lactated Ringer) are the fluids of choice for resuscitation.[46,48] There may be an association between hyperchloremia and acute kidney injury (AKI). When comparing high-chloride and low-chloride fluid strategies, critically ill patients in a chloride-restrictive group had more normal electrolyte and acid-base profiles and less incidence of AKI.[49,50] Although not substantiated in the horse, this may warrant consideration when planning a fluid strategy for horses with acute blood loss (**Table 1**).

Hypertonic saline is another useful crystalloid fluid that is available in 7.0% and 7.5% solutions. Low doses of hypertonic saline result in a rapid 2- to 4-fold expansion of the intravascular space, pulling fluid from the intracellular and interstitial spaces. Hypertonic saline is indicated for cases of moderate to severe acute hemorrhage whereby the source of blood loss is controlled. The recommended dose is 2 to 4 mL/kg (1–2 L for a 500-kg horse).

Colloids

Colloids are fluids composed of large molecules that are mostly retained within the intravascular space. Large intravascular concentrations help retain fluid within, and pull fluid into, the intravascular space. Colloids are indicated for rapid volume expansion in cases of moderate to severe hypovolemia. The usefulness of synthetic colloids (hydroxyethyl starch [HES]) in human medicine has been questioned due to potential side effects and associated mortality,[51,52] including allergic reactions, coagulopathies, and renal injury. These complications are dose related and more common among the higher-molecular-weight generations of HES.[51] A newer low-molecular-weight generation of HES has been recently evaluated in the horse and has similar benefits to the

Table 1
Composition of commonly used crystalloids used for resuscitative fluids

Fluid	Na^+ (mmol/L)	K^+ (mmol/L)	Ca^{2+} (mmol/L)	Mg^{2+} (mmol/L)	Cl^- (mmol/L)
Plasma	132–146	2.8–5.1	9.0–13	1.8–3	99–110
Plasma-Lyte A/Normosol R	140	5	0	3	98
Lactated Ringer	130	4	1.4	0	109
Acetated Ringer	130	5	1	1	112
0.9% Sodium	154	0	0	0	154

Data from Intravenous fluid therapy in adults in hospital. NICE clinical guideline 174. 2013. Last updated December 2016.

high-molecular-weight HES but with lower risk of accumulation in the circulation[53] and a more sustained effect on the colloid osmotic pressure with shorter duration of adverse effects on platelet function.[54,55] The recommended dose of HES is 5 to 10 mL/kg/d intravenously (IV), not to exceed 20 mg/kg/d.

Blood Products

Plasma is a naturally occurring colloid that is frequently used in critically ill hypovolemic patients. The advantage of using plasma over synthetic colloids is that it provides protein, antibodies, and clotting factors. The disadvantage of using plasma is reduced effectiveness in improving colloid oncotic pressure. Most plasma is frozen, requiring thawing before it can be used. In cases of acute blood loss, frozen plasma may not be the best choice for a resuscitation fluid.

Whole blood is also a colloid that exerts oncotic pressure and primarily stays within the intravascular space. Whole blood is indicated in many cases of hemorrhage, as RBCs and resultant oxygen carrying capacity and tissue oxygenation can be restored.

Determining a need to administer whole blood can be difficult, particularly if hemorrhage is confined to a body cavity. In cases of acute blood loss due to severe wounds, an estimation of blood loss is difficult and may be unobtainable depending on the circumstances of the trauma. In acute blood loss, assessment of physical parameters (tachycardia, dull, cool extremities, pale mucous membranes, and prolonged CRT) should be the minimum database used to estimate the degree of blood loss and the appropriate resuscitation fluid plan. It is important to remember that PCV and Total Solids (TS) are poor indicators of blood loss in the immediate (8–12 hour) posttrauma period.

Common general guidelines recommended for determining the need for whole blood include the following[43,46,56,57]:

- Estimated blood loss of greater than 30% (12–14 L)
- Clinical signs consistent with acute blood loss: tachycardia, tachypnea, pale mucous membranes, poor pulse quality
- Hyperlactatemia: $\geq$4 mmol/L (>2 mmol/L following fluid administration)
- Hematocrit of 18% to 20% in acute hemorrhage or 12% to 14% in chronic anemia
- Venous partial pressure of oxygen: if less than 30% to 35% suggests that peripheral tissues are oxygen starved and are pulling as much dissolved O_2 out of the blood as possible.

The amount of blood lost can be estimated using the following formula (this calculation should be performed once resuscitative crystalloids have been given and the PCV has had time to stabilize [8–12 hours])[46]:

- Blood lost (L) = [(PCV_{normal} – $PCV_{patient}$)/PCV_{normal}] · 0.08 · BW (kg)

Performing a Blood Transfusion

- Ideally, the blood donor horse should be blood typed and be negative for Aa and Qa alloantigens. In an emergency field situation, a blood-typed donor is usually not available. In that situation, a large healthy gelding, ideally of the same breed and greater than 500 kg, can be an ideal blood donor. Broodmares should not be considered as donors because of the possibility of possessing alloantibodies from pregnancy and foaling. Donkeys and mules have red blood cell (RBC) antigens and should also not be used for donors. If a horse needs a second transfusion, it is important that major and minor cross-matching be performed.

- How much blood needs to be collected? A replacement of 20% to 50% of the estimated loss is the goal. A donor can safely give up to 20% (15–18 mL/kg) of their blood volume per collection (7–9 L for a 500-kg donor).
  - Transfusion volume (L) = 0.1 · BW (kg) · [($PCV_{desired}$ − $PCV_{recipient}$)/PCV_{donor}]
- A large-bore catheter (10–12 gauge) should be aseptically placed in the donor jugular vein.
- Blood can be collected into sterile plastic bags or glass bottles. Collection into glass will cause inactivation of platelets. If the blood is to be transfused immediately following collection, acid-citrate dextrose can be used as the anticoagulant. If the blood is to be stored, citrate-phosphate-dextrose with adenine is recommended.
- For rapid collection, several techniques can be used. Occlude and distend the jugular veins by securing a roll of Elastikon (Johnson & Johnson, New Brunswick, NJ, USA) or a similar product, over each jugular vein distal to the catheter and secure in place. Suction can be applied to evacuated glass containers for large-volume collection. Place a second large-bore needle and collection set through the bottle seal and connect the set to a suction device. The suction will maintain a negative pressure within the bottle, increasing the rate of collection.
- The donor should receive 10 to 20 L of isotonic crystalloids during or immediately after blood collection. Donors should have a 30-day rest period between collections to regenerate erythrocytes.
- A filtered administration set should be used for the blood transfusion. Administration should be slow (2–10 mL/kg/h) for the first 20 to 30 minutes. If no adverse reaction is observed, the rate can be gradually increased to 20 mL/kg/h.
- Adverse reactions are as follows:
  - Attention to detail and careful collection and administration technique should be adhered to avoid non-immune-mediated adverse reactions such as sepsis.
  - Febrile, nonhemolytic reactions, allergic reactions, and hemolytic reactions are the most common adverse reactions.
  - Clinical signs common to febrile, nonhemolytic reactions include pyrexia and malaise. Treatment should include stopping transfusion administration or slowing the rate and treating with a nonsteroidal anti-inflammatory drug (NSAID) (flunixin meglumine, 1.1 mg/kg, IV).
  - Clinical signs common to allergic reactions include piloerection, pruritus, urticarial, and respiratory signs. Horses may also experience colic. Severe allergic reactions can progress to anaphylaxis and possible death. Treatment should include stopping the transfusion and administration of an antihistamine (diphenhydramine, 0.5–2.0 mg/kg, IV slowly or intramuscularly [IM]; hydroxyzine, 0.5–1.0 mg/kg, IM or orally) or a corticosteroid (prednisolone sodium succinate, 1 mg/kg, IV; dexamethasone, 0.05–0.1 mg/kg, IV or IM). In severe reactions, epinephrine can be given (0.01–0.02 mg/kg, IV or IM).
  - Clinical signs common to hemolytic reactions include hemoglobinemia, hemoglobinuria, tachycardia, tachypnea, fever, and restlessness. Treatment should include discontinuation of the transfusion and continued crystalloid administration. Hemolysis can be delayed and noted 3 to 5 days after transfusion administration.
- If multiple transfusions are required, it is imperative that major and minor cross-matching be performed for the donor and recipient. (See Mudge,[43] Magdesian,[46] and Hart[57]).

The author uses a combination of clinical signs and hematological data to determine the decision for blood transfusion. Horses with clinical signs of acute blood loss, including tachycardia, tachypnea, depression, and anorexia, are candidates for blood transfusion. Some clinicians use a PCV "cutoff" to determine whether a transfusion is necessary. In general, a PCV of 15% in combination with clinical signs of blood loss anemia should be treated with a blood transfusion. Once the decision for a blood transfusion has been made, the next consideration is selecting a suitable donor.

Additional Therapy

Additional therapy for horses suffering from severe traumatic wounds and excessive blood loss includes NSAID therapy and broad-spectrum antimicrobial therapy. It is also important to provide adequate nutritional support.[58]

DORSALLY LOCATED WOUNDS

Although wounds to the trunk normally do not result in substantial complications, they can become complicated if they are located over the dorsum of the horse because adequate ventral drainage is difficult to establish. Dorsal wounds are difficult to protect from contamination and secondary infection. Depending on the depth of the wound and the degree of contamination or infection, these wounds often dissect between tissue planes and can result in delayed or nonhealing wounds. Vacuum-assisted closure systems, or negative pressure wound therapy (NPWT), on large or deep productive dorsal wounds has been successful (**Fig. 9**). NPWT has been used extensively in human medicine and more recently in veterinary medicine, with only limited reports in the horse.[59–63] Primary use is in the management of infected wounds, in delayed wound healing, and as an aid in facilitating skin grafting.[64] NPWT can enhance wound healing with a combination of local immune modulation, mechanoreceptor stimulation, and hypoxia-mediated signaling, resulting in angiogenesis, extracellular matrix remodeling, and deposition of granulation tissue.[65,66] Establishing adequate sustained negative pressure can be difficult in the horse, but once established, a substantial

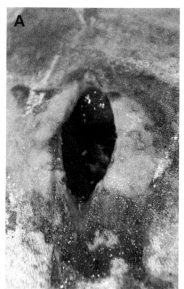 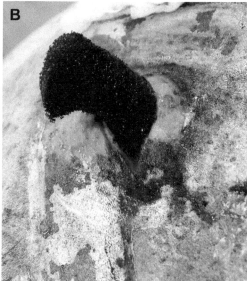

Fig. 9. (*A*) Dorsally located nonhealing wound due to bone sequestrum over S4. (*B*) Sequestrum was removed standing, and wound is packed with polyurethane foam in preparation for NPWT.

reduction in fluid production and wound healing time can occur. There are number of NPWT systems on the market today (**Table 2**).

For cases with financial constraints, a very affective and economical vacuum system can be manufactured with easily accessible materials (**Fig. 10**).

- Open cell polyurethane foam (acoustic grill foam) can be purchased in bulk. The bulk material can be cut into the desired sizes, packaged, and sterilized. The porosity of the foam is similar to the commercially available foam kits used for NPWT (400–600-μm pore size).
- Trim the foam to the appropriate size to fit within the margins of the wound.
- Using Metzenbaum scissors or a blade, create a narrow channel approximately 6 to 8 cm deep, splitting the thickness of the foam.
- Insert the tip of a red rubber catheter (28–34 French) into the channel.
- Prepare the skin surrounding the wound with acetone and apply a light coat of spray adhesive to the skin surrounding the wound, making sure the adhesive does not come into contact with the wound margins.
- Place the foam over the wound. If the wound is deep, the foam can be gently inserted into the wound.
- Apply an Ioban drape over the wound and 3 to 4 inches of the catheter, making sure the Ioban seals the entire circumference of the catheter. A second Ioban layer is often required to obtain an adequate seal.
- Using appropriate fittings, the catheter is affixed to a suction tubing and an IV coil. The line is suspended from the stall in such a way that the horse can move freely in the stall and lie down. The line is connected to a suction unit placed outside the stall. Small portable suction units are available that can be secured to the horse.

Table 2
Manufacturer/supplier of negative pressure wound therapy units

Manufacturer/Supplier	NPWT System
Acelity/KCI (SanAntonio, TX)	V.A.C. Therapy System
Mölnycke Health Care (Norcross, GA)	Avance Flex
4L Health (Huizhou, China)	Foryou NPWT Pro, Home, and Mini
Smith&Nephew (London, UK)	PICO RENASYS, RENASYS TOUCH, RENASYS EZ PLUS, and RENASYS GO
Cardinal Health (Innovative Therapies, Inc, Dublin, OH)	NRWT PRO and PRO to GO Kit, SVED
Hartman (Rock Hill, SC)	VivanoTec
Medela (McHenry, IL)	Invia Liberty and Invia Motion
ConvaTec	Avelle
Equinoxo2 Medical	UNI NPWT Foam Kit
Genadyne Biotechnologies, Inc (Hicksville, NY)	XLR8 and XLR8 Plus
H&R Healthcare (Lakewood, NJ)	UNO, Genadyne XLR8+, Prospera Por-II
Innovative Therapies (Cardinal Health, Inc)	NRWT PRO and PRO to GO Kit, SVED
Pensar Medical (Norco, CA)	Wound Pro
Alleva (Hong Kong)	extriCARE 2400, extriCARE 3600
Talley Group Ltd (St Albans, UK)	VENTURI Avanti, VENTURI compact, VENTURI Mino

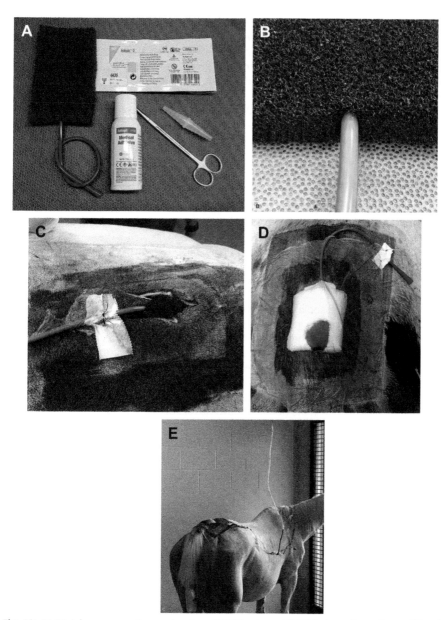

Fig. 10. Materials necessary to construct an NPWT system. (*A*) (1) Polyurethane foam, (2) red rubber catheter, (3) Ioban drape, (4) spray tissue adhesive, and (5) double Christmas tree style connector. (*B*) A small 6- to 8-cm channel is created in the foam for placement of a red rubber catheter. (*C*) The foam is loosely packed into the depths of the wound. The catheter can be secured to the skin to help prevent dislodging. (*D*) Sterile 4 × 4 gauze I placed over the wound. A light coat of spray adhesive is applied around the wound, and an Ioban drape is secured over the wound. Care is taken to assure that the Ioban is completely adhered around the catheter. (*E*) NPWT is active, and horse is able to move freely around stall and lie down.

The bandage over the NPWT should be removed, the wound assessed, and the system reapplied every 2 to 3 days. Leaving the bandage on longer can cause some discomfort on removal due to infiltration of granulation tissue into the foam. The NPWT is continued until a healthy granulation bed is present throughout the wound. If the wound remains exudative and does not have adequate drainage, the system can be left on longer. There is conflicting evidence as to the proper pressure setting to achieve the desired affects of NPWT. Currently the accepted standard pressure setting is −125 mm Hg. A recent study evaluated more than 1000 peer-reviewed articles looking at NPWT and came up with an acceptable therapeutic range of −40 mm Hg to −150 mm Hg.[67]

UROGENITAL WOUNDS

External trauma to the genitalia of the horse is not common. The most common genital trauma causing tissue damage in the mare is perineal body and rectovaginal (RV) tearing at the time of parturition. Stallions will occasionally sustain wounds to the penis and scrotum at the time of breeding or while making aggressive attempts to gain access to a mare for breeding.

Mare

RV injuries are often associated with mares that experience dystocia.[68] A 2005 retrospective study reported an incidence of 2.5% for RV trauma in a population of mares admitted for postpartum emergency.[68] In this study, 3 of the 4 mares that sustained RV injuries also had a history of prolapsed intestine (small intestine, rectum, and small colon) at the time of admission. RV tears are seen more commonly in well-muscled primiparous quarter horse mares and young nervous maiden mares that have excitable temperaments. Fetal malposition may also contribute to RV trauma.[69,70] A foal's foot may become entrapped in the dorsal transverse fold of the vestibulovaginal junction. If the foot is not repositioned either by retraction by the foal or assisted delivery, the foot can penetrate the tissues and result in varying degrees of tissue damage.

Classification of RV injuries[70]:

- First-degree RV laceration: the dorsal vestibule mucosa and skin of the dorsal commissure of the vulva are involved.
- Second-degree RV lacerations: the dorsal vestibule mucosa, submucosa, and muscles (constrictor vulvae) of the perineal body are involved.
- Third-degree RV laceration: complete disruption of the rectovestibular shelf, extending through the rectum, perineal body, and anal sphincter.
- RV fistula: penetration and disruption of the RV tissues without disruption of the perineal body.

Treatment

First-degree RV lacerations commonly do not require surgical manipulation. These lacerations heal well with supportive conservative wound care. A Caslicks procedure can help keep the tissue clean and reduce the need for open wound therapy.[70]

Second-degree RV lacerations do require surgical intervention to prevent the risk of future infection and infertility. The resultant muscle damage prevents normal function of the vulvar labia. If not repaired, these mares tend to develop poor perineal conformation and are predisposed to pneumovagina and urine pooling. If these wounds are noted immediately following parturition, they can be cleansed and successfully repaired. If the wounds are noted late (after 3–5 days), the wound should be treated as an open wound. Swelling and inflammation should subside and the wound edges should be allowed to epithelize. Delayed closure can be considered.[71] As soon as the wound is identified, the mare should be started on appropriate antimicrobial and NSAID therapy.

Third-degree RV lacerations are more complicated and can result in more postoperative complications due to tissue damage and contamination. Wound repair in the acute stage is not recommended because of extensive edema, trauma, and contamination. Repair at this stage is often unsuccessful. Third-degree lacerations should be managed as open wounds for 6 to 8 weeks to allow tissues to heal and scar tissue to remodel[70,71] (**Fig. 11**). Delaying repair until the foal is weaned can avoid exposure of the foal to a hospital environment and avoid the risk of altering lactation if diet changes are needed to manage the preoperative and postoperative period.[69]

Initial therapy should include wound management, vaginal hygiene, and supportive care of the mare. Because of the location of the wound, fecal contamination is unavoidable and persistent. The wound should be kept clean with frequent mild soap cleansing and tap water rinse. In some cases of severe trauma, debridement of devitalized tissues may be necessary. It is common with deep lacerations for fecal material to fall into the vagina. Keeping the vagina evacuated will help minimize gross contamination. Three to 5 days of NSAID therapy and 5 to 7 days of antimicrobial therapy are suggested for affected mares.[71,72]

Dietary management is very important in the overall success of RV laceration repair.[69–71] One to 2 weeks before the scheduled repair, a mare's diet should be altered to encourage soft feces. Lush green pasture is an excellent method to soften feces. Incorporating alfalfa, bran mashes, and/or pelleted diets into the diet, or administering laxatives, can also promote soft feces.

Methods of surgical repair of third-degree RV lacerations are described in numerous texts.[70–72] The most common method of repair (modified Goetze) is based on the Goetze (single-stage) and Aanes (2-stage) techniques. The method chosen is largely based on surgeon's preference. There have been several different techniques

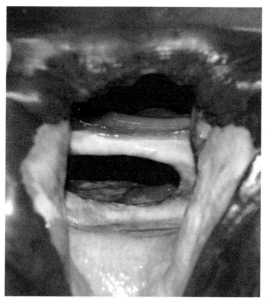

Fig. 11. Healed third-degree RV lacerations approximately 8 weeks after injury. Tissues are healed well and ready for repair. Note the fecal material in the vaginal vault.

reported recently describing different suturing techniques in the perineal tissues. One report described a transverse closure of the perineal tissues, thereby potentially reducing the reported postoperative complications of tenesmus, constipation, and repair failure.[73] In this report, all 8 repairs were successful with a 62.5% reported pregnancy rate the following season. Another report performed a 2-stage repair incorporating 3 parallel continuous circular suture lines, one centrally, and a second and third line abaxial to the central line. In this report, all 8 repairs healed well with a 71% reported pregnancy rate.[74] Two additional techniques described different suture patterns and pattern placement. One used an inside-out suture pattern to appose the vestibular flap followed by apposition of the rectal flap and perineal tissues simultaneously with the same suture pattern.[75] The second used a continuous horizontal mattress pattern in the vestibular flap, a Ford interlocking pattern in the perineal tissues, and a continuous horizontal mattress pattern in the rectal flap, similar to the modified Goetze technique.[76] All repairs using the inside-out technique healed well. At the time of the report, 3 of the 7 mares were bred and foaled without recurrence of a laceration; one was in foal, and 3 mares were in regular heat but not bred. In the Ford interlocking report, all repairs healed well except for one that developed an RV fistula that was successfully repaired. Of the 8 mares repaired and bred, 4 delivered normally without complications.

There are several factors that impact the successful repair of third-degree RV lacerations, including preoperative and postoperative diet management, the size of the injury, the amount of scar tissue present at the time of the repair, the amount of tension on the repair, and surgeon skill. The technique used should be based on surgeon's preference and comfort with the technique, and the technique that best suits the individual repair.

RV tear repair procedures are most commonly performed in the standing mare under epidural anesthesia (**Table 3**). Postoperatively, these mares should be maintained on NSAID and antimicrobial therapy as well as a fecal-softening diet. Potential complications of this procedure include dehiscence of the repair and the formation of an RV fistula.

Stallion/Gelding

Traumatic wounds to the male genitalia are not common and are most often seen in breeding stallions due to their activity and behavior. Stallions, and some geldings, can traumatize the penis and/or testicles during an act of breeding or attempted breeding. This trauma can occur from direct kicks from a mare or inaccurate intromission. With an erect or exposed penis, the stallion or gelding may come into contact with fencing, brush, or other objects.[77] Clean fresh wounds to the penis or prepuce can be debrided and closed primarily.

Table 3 Common local anesthetics used for standing caudal epidural anesthesia				
Drug	Dose (mg/kg)	Onset of Action (min)	Duration of Action	Recommended Volume (mL)
Lidocaine 2%	0.2–0.35	5–15	60–90 min	5–8
Mepivacaine	0.2–0.25	6–10	90–120 min	5–8
Xyalazine + Local	0.17 0.22	15	4–6 h	5–8

From Natalini CC, Driessen B. Epidural and spinal anesthesia and analgesia in the equine. Clin Tech Equine Pract 2007;6:145–53; with permission.

Penile and scrotal wounds can be complicated because of the dependent location. With most penile trauma, with or without a wound, the inflammation and swelling result in pain, extension of the penis, and progressive dependent edema and impaired venous and lymphatic drainage. With the increase in size, weight, and pain associated with genital trauma, an affected horse can lose the ability to retract the penis due to retractor muscle fatigue, resulting in paraphimosis, or the inability to retract the penis into the prepuce. Prolonged environmental exposure can predispose to further damage.[77] These traumas are true emergencies, especially in breeding stallions.

Therapy is focused on reducing swelling, supporting the penis, and reestablishing normal function as soon as possible. The penis and scrotum should be examined very closely for evidence of urethral involvement or involvement of the cavernous tissues along the shaft of the penis and any penetrating wounds to the scrotum resulting in testicular injury. If the urethra is involved and there are concerns with urination, rectal palpation to evaluate the bladder and urinary catheterization are indicated. If there is severe damage to the urethra, performing a temporary perineal urethrostomy should be considered.

Controlling inflammation and edema is crucial in cases of penile trauma to reduce complications of muscle fatigue and nerve damage. Systemic anti-inflammatories and local therapy, including hydrotherapy, massage, application of a compressive wrap or pneumatic pressure bag,[78] and topical glycerin, can aid in reducing edema[79] (**Fig. 12**). An ointment commonly used for penile wounds in bulls can work well in horses (Petercillin [petrolatum, tetracycline, and scarlet oil]). When edema has been reduced, attempts should be made to place the penis into the prepuce and secure in place by placing a purse-string suture at the preputial orifice, drawing it down to where 1 to 2 fingers can be placed through the orifice. A modified Buhner suture technique has also been described.[80] An alternative to a purse-string suture or Buhner stitch is application of a probang device.[81] The probang device is an atraumatic penile repulsion device that is constructed out of readily available materials[81]:

- Two-inch PVC tubing cut to 15 to 25 inches
- Appropriate diameter endotracheal or nasogastric tube (fits snuggly into internal diameter of PVC tubing)
- Roll cotton
- One pair of large latex gloves
- Nitrofurazone ointment
- Four to 6 rolls of Elastikon
- One roll of white adhesive tape

The probang device is placed into the preputial sheath preventing the penis from prolapsing.

If the penis cannot be replaced into the prepuce, a suspensory sling should be implemented. A sling should be made out of a mesh material to allow free passage of urine. The mesh is cut to a size that will allow adequate and complete support of the penis. Rubber tubing, or a similar material, is attached to the front and back of the mesh material. The front tubing is tied over the back of the horse, and the back tubing is extended through the back legs, brought over the tail, and secured to the front tubing.[79] Aggressive therapy should continue until the penis can be replaced into the preputial sheath.

Wound management should continue with debridement of any devitalized tissue. The penis is difficult to bandage but can be done if necessary as long as it is supported. If the penis can be placed into the sheath, bandaging is not needed. Broad-spectrum antimicrobial therapy should be initiated and continued until granulation of the wound occurs.

Clean lacerations of the shaft of the penis can be closed primarily. It is essential the wound be evaluated thoroughly in order to determine what tissues are involved.

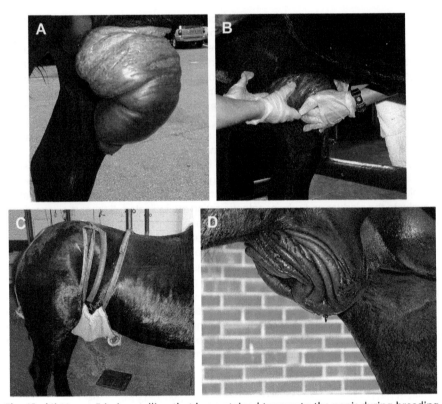

Fig. 12. (A) Young Friesian stallion that has sustained trauma to the penis during breeding. The penis cannot be retracted in the preputial sheath. (B) The swollen penis is being massaged to help reduce the edema. (C) A sling has been constructed out of a mesh material to allow free passage of urine. (D) Following 2 days of aggressive therapy, the stallion can now retract the penis into the preputial sheath.

Disruption of the tunica albuginea, corpus cavernosum, and urethral tissue must be dealt with individually and closed appropriately in order to prevent hemorrhage and reestablish normal function.[82] Deep wounds to the shaft of the penis can cause scarring and urethral stricture requiring surgical intervention. If the penis must be maintained in the prepuce, a permanent perineal urethrostomy can be performed. If the horse is unable to completely retract the penis into the prepuce and normal urinary function is desired, a partial phallectomy can be performed proximal to the compromised tissue. Multiple partial phallectomy techniques are described, including the Scott, Williams, and the Vinsot.[82,83] If the trauma extends proximal to the internal lamina of the prepuce, en bloc resection of the penis with preputial ablation may be required in combination with a permanent perineal urethrostomy[82,84,85] (**Fig. 13**).

Wounds to the prepuce can be closed primarily, or heal by second intention. Scar tissue can prevent the normal telescoping function of the prepuce and require segmental posthioplasty (reefing) to restore normal function.[82]

SUMMARY

Wound management in the horse is often straightforward and uncomplicated. However, because of horses' size, curious nature, and fight-or-flight reaction to noxious

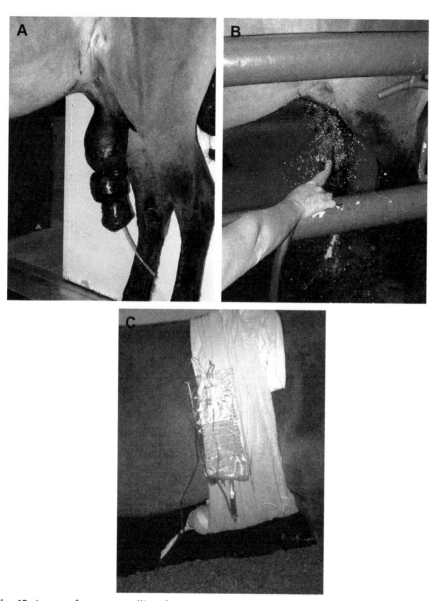

Fig. 13. Image of a young stallion that attempted to jump out of a stall to gain access to a mare. The erect penis became hung in the stall door. (*A*) Note the severe swelling and discoloration of the penis. A urinary catheter was placed due to the inability to urinate. (*B*) Horse in (*A*) was treated with hydrotherapy multiple times a day. (*C*) Penis was placed in a pressure bandage and secured to the ventral abdomen. Urine was collected to monitor urine output. This horse went on to necrosis and sloughed most of his penis. Once the tissues started to granulate, the horse was taken to surgery for a partial phallectomy with preputial ablation.

stimuli, many wounds are associated with substantial tissue injury and loss and high-impact trauma. In managing complicated wounds, it is imperative to have an excellent working knowledge of anatomy and the processes of wound healing. Being diligent and complete in the assessment of these patients and their wounds as well as the diagnostic workup and therapeutic planning can help manage these complicated wounds. Taking the approach of "Assume the worst until proven otherwise" can help reduce the risk of a missed diagnosis.

REFERENCES

1. Dart AJ, Sole-Guitart A, Stashak TS, et al. Selected factors that negatively impact healing. In: Theoret CL, Schumacher J, editors. Equine wound management. 3rd edition. Ames (IA): Wiley-Blackwell; 2016. p. 30–46.
2. Clem MF, DeBowes RM, Yovich JV, et al. Osseous sequestration in the horse a review of 68 cases. Vet Surg 1988;17(1):2–5.
3. Schwartz AJ, Wilson DA, Keegan KG, et al. Factors regulating collagen synthesis and degradation during second-intention healing of wounds in the thoracic region and the distal aspect of the forelimb of horses. Am J Vet Res 2002;63:1564–70.
4. Theoret CL, Barber SM, Moyana TN, et al. Expression of transforming growth factor ß1, ß3, and basic fibroblast growth factor in full-thickness skin wounds of equine limbs and thorax. Vet Surg 2001;30:269–77.
5. Theoret CL, Barber SM, Moyana TN, et al. Preliminary observations on expression of transforming growth factors ß1 and ß3 in equine full-thickness skin wounds healing normally or with exuberant granulation tissue. Vet Surg 2002;31:266–73.
6. Celeste CJ, Deschene K, Riley CB, et al. Regional differences in wound oxygenation during normal healing in an equine model of cutaneous fibroproliferative disorder. Wound Repair Regen 2010;19:89–97.
7. Wilmink JM, Stolk PWT, van Weeren PR, et al. Differences in second-intention wound healing between horses and ponies: macroscopical aspects. Equine Vet J 1999;31:53–60.
8. Wilmink JM, van Weeren PR, Stolk PW, et al. Differences in second-intention wound healing between horses and ponies: histological aspects. Equine Vet J 1999;31:61–7.
9. Post EM, Singer ER, Clegg PD, et al. Retrospective study of 24 cases of septic calcaneal bursitis in the horse. Equine Vet J 2003;35(7):662–8.
10. Whitcomb MB. Ultrasonography of the equine tarsus. Proc Am Assoc Equine Pract 2006;52:13–30.
11. Jacobs KA, Leach DH, Fretz PB, et al. Comparative aspects of the healing of excisional wounds on the leg and body of horses. Vet Surg 1984;13:83.
12. Theoret CL, Wilmink JM. Aberrant wound healing in the horse: naturally occurring conditions reminiscent of those observed in man. Wound Repair Regen 2013;21:365–71.
13. Hanson RR, Schumacher J. Degloving injuries of the distal aspect of the limb. In: Theoret CL, Schumacher J, editors. Equine wound management. 3rd edition. Ames (IA): Wiley-Blackwell; 2016. p. 352.
14. Hanson R. Complications of equine wound management and dermatologic surgery. Vet Clin North Am Equine Pract 2009;24:663–96.
15. Hendrix SM, Baxter GM. Management of complicated wounds. Vet Clin North Am Equine Pract 2005;21:217–30.
16. Richardson DW, Ahern BJ. Synovial and osseous infections. In: Auer AA, Stick AA, editors. Equine surgery. 4th edition. St Louis (MO): Elsevier-Saunders; 2012. p. 1189–201.
17. Booth TM, Knottenbelt DC. Distal limb casts in equine wound management. Equine Vet Educ 1999;11(5):273–80.

18. Dart AJ, Guitart AS, Stashak TS, et al. Management practices that influence wound infection and healing. In: Theoret CL, Schumacher J, editors. Equine wound management. 3rd edition. Ames (IA): Wiley-Blackwell; 2016. p. 47–74.
19. Edlich RF, Rodeheaver GT, Thacker JG. Revolutionary advances in the management of traumatic wounds in the emergency department during the last 40 years: Part 1. J Emerg Med 2010;38(1):40–50.
20. Schultz GS, Sibbald RG, Falanga V, et al. Wound bed preparation: a systematic approach to wound management. Wound Repair Regen 2003;11:1–28.
21. Stashak TS, Schumacher J. Principles and techniques for reconstructive surgery. In: Theoret CL, Schumacher J, editors. Equine wound management. 3rd edition. Ames (IA): Wiley-Blackwell; 2016. p. 200.
22. Provost PJ, Bailey JV. Principles of plastic reconstructive surgery. In: Auer AA, Stick AA, editors. Equine surgery. 4th edition. St Louis (MO): Elsevier-Saunders; 2012. p. 271–84.
23. Theoret CL, Wilmink JM. Exuberant granulation tissue. In: Theoret CL, Schumacher J, editors. Equine wound management. 3rd edition. Ames (IA): Wiley-Blackwell; 2016. p. 369–87.
24. Theoret CL, Wilmink JM. Treatment of exuberant granulation tissue. In: Stashak TS, Theoret CL, editors. Equine wound management. 2nd edition. Ames (IA): Wiley-Blackwell; 2008. p. 445–62.
25. Gillespie Harmon CC, Hawkins JF, Li J, et al. Effects of topical application of silver sulfadiazine cream, triple antimicrobial ointment, or hyperosmolar nanoemulsion on wound healing, bacterial load, and exuberant granulation tissue formation in bandaged full-thickness equine skin wounds. Am J Vet Res 2017;78:638–46.
26. Dahlgren LA, Milton SC, Boswell SG. Evaluation of a hyaluronic acid-based biomaterial to enhance wound healing in the equine distal limb. J Equine Vet Sci 2016;44:90–9.
27. Berry DB, Sullins KE. Effects of topical application of antimicrobials and bandaging on healing and granulation tissue formation in wounds of the distal aspect of the limbs in horses. Am J Vet Res 2003;64:88–92.
28. Dart AJ, Perkins NR, Dart CM, et al. Effect of bandaging on second intention healing of wounds of the distal limb in horses. Aust Vet J 2009;87(6):215–8.
29. Lepault E, Celeste C, Dore M, et al. Comparative study on microvascular occlusion and apoptosis in body and limb wounds in the horse. Wound Repair Regen 2005;13:520–9.
30. Fretz PB, Martin GS, Jacobs KA, et al. Treatment of exuberant granulation tissue in the horse evaluation of four methods. Vet Surg 1983;12(3):137–40.
31. Carney SA, Cason CG, Gower JP, et al. Cica-Care gel sheeting in the management of hypertrophic scarring. Burns 1994;20:163–7.
32. Gold MH, Foster TD, Adair MA, et al. Prevention of hypertrophic scars and keloids by the prophylactic use of topical silicone gel sheets following a surgical procedure in an office setting. Dermatol Surg 2001;27:641–4.
33. Momeni M, Hafezi F, Rahbar H, et al. Effects of silicone gel on burn scars. Burns 2009;35:70–4.
34. Ducharme-Desjarlais M, Celeste CJ, Lepault E. Effect of a silicon-containing dressing on exuberant granulation tissue formation and wound repair on horses. Am J Vet Res 2005;66:1133–9.
35. Hackett RP. How to prevent and treat exuberant granulation tissue. Proc Am Assoc Equine Pract 2011;57:367–73.
36. Barber SM. Second intention wound healing in the horse: the effect of bandages and topical corticosteroids. Proc Am Assoc Equine Pract 1990;35:107–16.

37. Sullivan TP, Eaglstein WH, Davis SC, et al. The pig as a model for human wound healing. Wound Repair Regen 2001;9:66–76.
38. Marks JG, Cano C, Leitzel K, et al. Inhibition of wound healing by topical steroids. J Dermatol Surg Oncol 1983;9(10):819–21.
39. Wilmink JM, van Weeren PR. A second-intention repair in the horse and pony and management of exuberant granulation tissue. Vet Clin North Am Equine Pract 2005;21:15–32.
40. Knottenbelt DC. A suggested clinical classification for the equine sarcoid. Clin Tech Equine Pract 2005;4:278–95.
41. Knottenbelt DC. Equine wound management: are there significant differences in healing at different sites on the body? Vet Dermatol 1997;8:273–90.
42. Jann H, Pasquini C. Wounds of the distal limb complicated by involvement of deep structures. Vet Clin North Am Equine Pract 2005;21:145–65.
43. Mudge MC. Acute hemorrhage and blood transfusions in horses. Vet Clin North Am Equine Pract 2014;30:427–36.
44. Barber SM. Management of wounds to the neck and body. In: Theoret CL, Schumacher J, editors. Equine wound management. 3rd edition. Ames (IA): Wiley-Blackwell; 2016. p. 280.
45. Carr EA. Shock: pathophysiology, diagnosis, treatment, and physiologic response to trauma. In: Auer AA, Stick AA, editors. Equine surgery. 4th edition. St Louis (MO): Elsevier-Saunders; 2012. p. 1–13.
46. Magdesian KG. Acute blood loss. Compend Contin Educ Pract Vet 2008;3:80–90.
47. Vincent JL, Backer DD. Circulatory shock. N Engl J Med 2013;369:1726–34.
48. Fielding L. Crystalloid and colloid therapy. Vet Clin North Am Equine Pract 2014;30:415–25.
49. Yunos N, Bellomo R, Hedgarty C, et al. Association between a chloride-liberal vs chloride-restrictive intravenous fluid administration strategy and kidney injury in critically ill adults. J Am Med Assoc 2012;308:1566–672.
50. Sen A, Keener CM, Sileanu FE, et al. Chloride content of fluids used for large-volume resuscitation is associated with reduced survival. Crit Care Med 2017;2:146–53.
51. Cazzolli D, Prittie J. The crystalloid-colloid debate: consequences of resuscitation fluid selection in veterinary critical care. J Vet Emer Crit Care (San Antonio) 2015;25(1):6–19.
52. Neto AS, Veelo DP, Peireira VG, et al. Fluid resuscitation with hydroxyethyl starches in patients with sepsis is associated with an increased incidence of acute kidney injury and use of renal replacement therapy: a systemic review and meta-analysis of the literature. J Crit Care 2014;29:185.e1–7.
53. Epstein KL, Bergren A, Nie B, et al. Comparison of the pharmacokinetics of two formulations of hydroxyethyl starch in healthy horses. J Vet Pharmacol Ther 2016;40:309–13.
54. Epstein KL, Bergren A, Giguere S, et al. Cardiovascular, colloid osmotic pressure, and hemostatic effects of 2 formulations of hydroxyethyl starch in healthy horses. J Vet Intern Med 2014;28:223–33.
55. Viljoen A, Page PC, Fosgate GT, et al. Coagulation, oncotic and haemodilutional effects of a third-generation hydroxyethyl starch (130/0.3) solution in horses. Equine Vet J 2014;46:739–44.
56. Cook VL, Southwood LL. Fluid therapy. In: Southwood LL, Wilkins PA, editors. Equine emergency and critical care medicine. Boca Raton (FL): CRC Press, Taylor & Francis Group; 2015. p. 653–74.

57. Hart KA. Blood transfusions and transfusion reactions. In: Sprayberry KA, Robinson NE, editors. Robinson's current therapy in equine medicine. 7th edition. St Louis (MO): Elsevier-Saunders; 2015. p. 484–9.

58. Carr EA, Holcombe SJ. Nutrition of critically ill horses. Vet Clin North Am Equine Pract 2009;25:93–108.

59. Florczyk A, Rosser J. Negative pressure wound therapy as management of a chronic distal limb wound in the horse. J Equine Vet Sci 2017;55:9–11.

60. Van Hecke LL, Haspeslagh M, Hermans K, et al. Comparison of antibacterial effects among three foams used with negative pressure wound therapy in an ex vivo equine perfused wound model. Am J Vet Res 2016;77(12):1325–31.

61. Jordana M, Pint E, Martens A. The use of vacuum-assisted wound closure to enhance skin graft acceptance in a horse. Vlaams Diergeneeskundig Tijdschrift 2011;80:343–50.

62. Gemeinhardt KD, Molnar JA. Vacuum-assisted closure for management of a traumatic neck wound in a horse. Equine Vet Educ 2005;17(1):27–33.

63. Rettig MJ, Lischer CJ. Treatment of chronic septic osteoarthritis of the antebrachiocarpal joint with a synovial-cutaneous fistula utilizing arthroscopic lavage combined with ultrasonic assisted wound therapy and vacuum assisted closure with a novel wound lavage system. Equine Vet Educ 2017;29(1):27–32.

64. Orsini JA, Elce Y, Kraus B. Management of severely infected wounds in the equine patient. Clin Tech Equine Pract 2004;3:225–36.

65. Stanley BJ. Negative pressure wound therapy. Vet Clin North Am Small Anim Pract 2017;47:1203–20.

66. Glass GE, Murphy GF, Esmaeili A, et al. Systemic review of molecular mechanism of action of negative-pressure wound therapy. Br J Surg 2014;101:1627–36.

67. Birke-Sorensen H, Malmsjo M, Rome P, et al. Evidence-based recommendations for negative pressure wound therapy: treatment variables (pressure levels, wound filler and contact layer) - Steps towards an international consensus. J Plast Reconstr Aesthet Sur 2011;64:S1–16.

68. Dolente BA, Sullivan EK, Boston R. Mares admitted to a referral hospital for postpartum emergencies: 163 cases (1992-2002). J Vet Emerg Crit Care 2005;15(3): 193–200.

69. LeBlanc MM. Common peripartum problems in the mare. J Equine Vet Sci 2008; 28(11):709–15.

70. Woodie JB. Vulva, vestibule, vagine, and cervix. In: Auer AA, Stick AA, editors. Equine surgery. 4th edition. St Louis (MO): Elsevier-Saunders; 2012. p. 866–83.

71. Moll HD, Slone DE. Perineal lacerations and rectovestibular fistulas. In: Wolfe DF, Moll HD, editors. Large animal urogenital surgery. Baltimore (MD): Williams & Wilkins; 1999. p. 103–8.

72. Trotter GW. Surgery of the perineum in the mare. In: McKinnon AO, Voss JL, editors. Equine reproduction. Media (PA): Williams & Wilkins; 1993. p. 417–27.

73. Kasikci G, Horoz H, Alkan S, et al. A modified surgical technique for repairing third-degree perineal lacerations in mares. Acta Vet Hung 2005;53(2):257–64.

74. Climent F, Ribera T, Arguelles, et al. Modified technique for the repair of third-degree rectovaginal lacerations in mares. Vet Rec 2009;164:393–6.

75. Anand A, Singh SS. Inside-out continuous suturing technique for the repair of third-degree perineal lacerations in mares. J Equine Vet Sci 2015;35:147–52.

76. Mosbah E. A modified one-stage repair of third-degree rectovestibular lacerations in mares. J Equine Vet Sci 2012;32:211–5.

77. Perkins NR, Frazer GS. Reproductive emergencies in the stallion. Vet Clin North Am Equine Pract 1994;10(3):671–83.

78. Brouwer ED, Ribera T, Climent F, et al. Alternative method to facilitate resolution of paraphimosis after penile trauma in the horse. Equine Vet Educ 2017;29(12): 655–8.

79. Brinsko SP, Blanchard TL, Varner DD. How to treat paraphimosis. Proc Am Assoc Equine Pract 2007;53:580–2.

80. Aurich JE, Aurich C. Treatment of penile prolapse in horses using a modified Büh-ner suture technique. Vet Rec 2006;159:491–2.

81. Koch C, O'Brien T, Livesey MA. How to construct and apply a penile repulsion device (Probang) to manage paraphimosis. Proc Am Assoc Equine Pract 2009; 55:338–41.

82. Schumacher J. Penis and prepuce. In: Auer AA, Stick AA, editors. Equine sur-gery. 4th edition. St Louis (MO): Elsevier-Saunders; 2012. p. 840–66.

83. Arnold CE, Brinsko SP, Love CC, et al. Use of a modified Vinsot technique for par-tial phallectomy in 11 standing horses. J Am Vet Med Assoc 2010;237:82–6.

84. Doles J, Williams JW, Yarbrough TB. Penile amputation and sheath ablation in the horse. Vet Surg 2001;30:327.

85. Wylie CE, Payne RJ. A modified technique for penile amputation and preputial ablation in the horse. Equine Vet Educ 2016;28(5):269–75.

Nonhealing Wounds of the Equine Limb

Michael Maher, DVM, Leann Kuebelbeck, DVM*

KEYWORDS

- Nonhealing wound • Chronic wound • Exuberant granulation tissue

KEY POINTS

- Horses present a unique challenge with regard to wound healing, particularly in the distal limb.
- Treating the nonhealing wound requires assessment of the general health of the horse.
- Successful resolution of a nonhealing wound requires resolution of the underlying inflammation/infection.
- Wound débridement is the mainstay to resolution of the underlying inflammation/infection.
- Additional therapies (wound closure, wound dressings, and skin grafts) can facilitate healing.

INTRODUCTION

Chronic (nonhealing) wounds are those that fail to proceed through the normal stages of wound healing in an orderly and timely fashion. Due to circumstances commonly encountered when horses are wounded, nonhealing wounds are a challenge all equine practitioners face. An understanding of why horses develop nonhealing wounds and options for management of this condition helps ease some of the frustration.

Wound Healing

Three stages of wound healing include the inflammatory stage, the proliferation stage, and finally the maturation/remodeling stage.[1] There are unique factors of wound healing in the horse that have a negative impact on these stages. First, there are differences in wound healing among equine species. Ponies heal better than horses due to horses mounting a weaker but more prolonged inflammatory stage. This inefficient inflammatory stage is believed to make the wound more susceptible to infection as well as contribute to a prolonged proliferative stage of healing. Second, the rate of healing varies by the location of wounds, with wounds on the main body healing

Disclosure Statement: None.
Brandon Equine Medical Center, 605 East Bloomingdale Avenue, Brandon, FL 33511, USA
* Corresponding author.
E-mail address: lkuebelbeck@brandonequine.com

more quickly than distal limb wounds.[2–6] Distal limb wounds tend to be in areas of higher motion, have less soft tissue coverage, are more prone to infection, and tend to develop excessive granulation tissue (EGT). Because distal limb wounds inherently have less skin to mobilize for wound repair, wound orientation in relation to skin tension lines plays a role in the healing process. Although the lines of skin tension have not been fully investigated in the horse, it has been suggested that the lines of the skin color pattern in tigers and zebras resemble the orientation of skin tension lines in the dog. In the absence of definitive information regarding skin tension lines in the horse, this same generality is used when planning reconstructive procedures in the horse and also provides a template of the tensile forces placed on distal limb skin wounds of horses. Those wounds that occur parallel to lines of tension have less gap than those wounds that occur at right angles (large gap) or oblique angles (curvilinear gap) to the maximal lines of tension.[6–8]

Fibroplasia, or the formation of granulation tissue, has many important functions, which change continuously through the healing process. Granulations tissue fills wound defects in the early stages, forms a barrier against external contaminants, provides myofibroblasts for wound contraction, and forms the subcutaneous tissue bed over which epithelium can migrate. Ideally granulation tissue only fills the wound and then contraction and epithelialization occur to complete healing. In many distal limb wounds, however, proliferation is prolonged, resulting in the formation of EGT.[9–11] The classic clinical sign of EGT is the protrusion of tissue above the surrounding skin wound margin.

Presentation of Nonhealing Wounds

Nonhealing wounds in equine patients typically present in 3 different ways:

1. Wounds that do not heal because of local infection secondary to bone sequestrum, underlying necrotic tendon or ligament, or a residual foreign body that was acquired when the wound occurred.

    These wounds typically have some degree of EGT. Frequently these wounds will be irregular and contain cracks or clefts which often can be followed to the source of the local infection/inflammation.

2. Wounds that have arrested healing and have become dry, chronic wounds.

    These wounds do not have EGT and frequently need stimulation to proceed with the formation of granulation tissue.

3. Chronic cases of EGT on the distal limb that have resulted in large, raised masses.

    The EGT is usually very fibrous and is nourished by large blood vessels and frequently is innervated to some degree.

PATIENT EVALUATION OVERVIEW
Comprehensive Physical Examination

It is easy to get distracted by the presence of a wound and neglect to look at the patient as a whole. One of the first steps when evaluating a nonhealing wound is to perform a complete physical examination and evaluate the patient for existing comorbidities. Any such issues should be addressed as quickly as possible. In older horses, this may involve addressing pituitary pars intermedia dysfunction or equine metabolic syndrome, among other issues. Management of common endocrine conditions often includes a combination of exercise, dietary modification, and possibly thyroid supplementation or pergolide, depending on which condition is treated. The Equine Endocrinology Group has provided good guidelines for diagnosing and treating such issues in the authors' equine patients.[12]

Wound Evaluation

After physical examination of the patient, the wound should be evaluated to help identify reasons for nonhealing. The location and size of the wound should be noted. Signs of wound infection include evidence of inflammation, edematous granulation tissue, discolored granulation tissue, draining tracts, and odor and should lead the practitioner into further diagnostics.[7]

Digital exploration of the wound should be performed to help identify a cause for delayed healing and sources of underlying infection. Common causes include bony sequestrum, foreign body, and necrotic tendon/ligament.

If infection is suspected, culture and sensitivity should be obtained to help direct antimicrobial therapy. Although not routinely performed in a clinical setting, a quantitative bacterial count can be used to confirm true infection of the wound. Radiographs are useful in identifying bony sequestrum or other radiodense foreign bodies (**Fig. 1**). Positive contrast fistulograms can be performed to help identify radiolucent foreign bodies. Ultrasonography can also be useful in identifying foreign bodies not detected with radiography. Potential abnormalities of the wound bed, such as sarcoids, neoplasia, or habronemiasis, can be identified by histopathology and should be considered when dealing with a chronic, nonhealing wound that is not responding to typical therapies.

PHARMACOLOGIC TREATMENT OPTIONS
Antimicrobial Therapy

Systemic antibiotics have value in treating some nonhealing wounds, but many of the chronic nonhealing wounds practitioners deal with are amenable to topical or regional

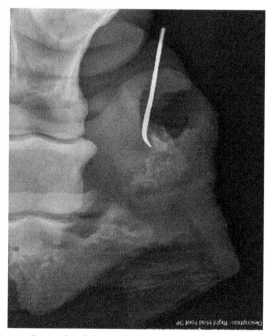

Fig. 1. Dorsoplantar radiograph of the right hind foot with a chronically infected lateral collateral cartilage of the distal phalanx. The hemostat followed an external draining tract.

antimicrobials. While appropriate antimicrobial therapies should be instituted when pathogenic bacteria resulting in infection are present in a nonhealing wound, often of greater importance is the débridement/excision of infected tissues (necrotic tendon/ligament, bone sequestra, or foreign body removal). Those cases that require systemic antimicrobials should have therapy based on culture and sensitivity results whenever possible.

Corticosteroid Therapy

Topical corticosteroid application for management of EGT has been described. Corticosteroids can have a detrimental effect on wound healing, so administration should be limited to 1 to 2 treatments.[13–15]

NONPHARMACOLOGIC TREATMENT OPTIONS
Bandaging

Nearly all nonhealing wounds of the distal limb are treated with some form of bandaging, especially after surgical débridement is performed. Bandages, casts, and external support are covered extensively in another article, so are addressed briefly (see Randy B. Eggleston's article, "Equine Wound Management: Bandages, Casts, and External Support," in this issue).

Wounds that have arrested healing in the early stages and are dry with minimal to no granulation tissue may best be bandaged with a product that stimulates the healing cascade. This often can be achieved using hydrophilic dressings. These dressings include naturally occurring products from a range of polysaccharide materials, such as dextranomers, alginates, freeze-dried gels, and chitin.[14] Of these, a calcium alginate dressing (Curasorb or Nu-Derm, Smith and Nephew, Inc, Andover (MA)) that is hydrated with saline may be the best choice to start the healing cascade and initiate granulation tissue development. When moistened with saline, the initial dry felt-like material creates a hydrophilic gel on the wound surface that forms via a calcium and sodium ion exchange, thus providing a moist environment conducive to wound healing.[15] A semiocclusive nonadherent pad should be placed over the calcium alginate dressing followed by a secondary and tertiary bandage layer.

Bandaging of a nonhealing wound that features exuberant granulation tissue is straightforward. After the EGT has been débrided (described later), a hemostatic compression bandage is placed initially and then replaced 12 hours to 24 hours later with a silicone gel dressing (occlusive synthetic bandage, such as Cica-Care), which promotes moist wound healing. Silicone gel dressings can prevent exuberant granulation tissue in experimentally created equine limb wounds.[16] Silicone gel dressings are marketed in the human field for treatment of wound overhealing (hypertrophic scar and keloid), with great success.[17–19] These dressings are fully occlusive and seem to occlude microvessels on the wound surface and gradually decrease oxygen tension in the tissues until a point of anoxia, when fibroblasts can no longer function and undergo apoptosis. The ratio of collagen synthesis to degradation is then altered in favor of the latter, thus minimizing fibrosis.[20]

Hyperbaric Oxygen Therapy

Hyperbaric oxygen therapy has been used in human and veterinary medicine for management of chronic wounds. Although some human studies have found its use to decrease wound edema, increase tissue oxygenation, and improve antimicrobial activity, similar results have not been demonstrated in the horse.[21] Further research is warranted for hyperbaric oxygen therapy in horses (see R. Reid Hanson's article, "Medical Therapy in Equine Wound Management," in this issue).

Biological and Regenerative Therapies

Many biological dressings and topical regenerative therapies have been evaluated (see Britta S. Leise's article, "Topical Wound Medications," and Linda A. Dahlgren's article, "Regenerative Medicine Therapies for Equine Wound Management," in this issue).

COMBINATION THERAPIES

It is safe to say that essentially all therapies for nonhealing wounds are used in various combinations because no single treatment is completely therapeutic as a single modality.

SURGICAL TREATMENT OPTIONS
Débridement

Management of a nonhealing wound inevitably involves some form of débridement. Although acute wounds, or occasional early chronic wounds, may lend themselves to enzymatic débridement (a collagenase product), biodébridement (maggots), or autolytic débridement (hydrogels or hydrocolloid dressings), a nonhealing wound almost always requires physical débridement using a scalpel blade, curette, or some other sharp instrument. Although various dressings and topical treatments have an important role in various stages of wound healing, such therapies do not likely mitigate the need for débridement of a chronic wound. Regardless of the method used, effective débridement of chronic wounds is accepted as an essential component of care throughout the wound healing continuum.[22]

After any chronic inflammatory process has been addressed (sequestrum removal, necrotic tendon/ligament débridement, foreign body extraction, and so forth), all EGT that protrudes above the wound margins should be excised with care not to damage newly migrating epithelium at the wound margins. Débridement needs to be repeated if/when the granulation tissue protrudes again above the wound margin. After débridement, a pressure bandage should be applied for 12 hours to 24 hours, followed by the application of a dressing, such as the silicone gel.

Horses with chronic, large masses of fibroplastic tissue on the distal limbs may require general anesthesia to excise the EGT because not only are these masses well vascularized but also many of them are at least partially innervated and may be difficult to desensitize with local anesthesia (**Fig. 2**). When chronic granulation tissue and fibroplasia are debulked, surrounding normal haired skin is difficult to elevate. There is typically strong adherence to the underlying dysplastic tissue, and this skin has minimal elasticity. Therefore, delayed primary closure is difficult and a large open wound is usually the end result (**Fig. 3**). In these situations, skin grafting is the best option to try to achieve epithelialization of these chronic wounds after aggressive débridement.

Wound Closure

Ideally, a chronic wound is sharply débrided and converted into an acute wound, which lends itself to primary closure. For this to be successful, there needs to be minimal bacterial contamination, minimal loss of tissue, and minimal tension of the closure site.[1] These criteria are difficult to achieve on the distal limbs of horses. Therefore, there are several additional methods to help facilitate wound resolution (see Louis

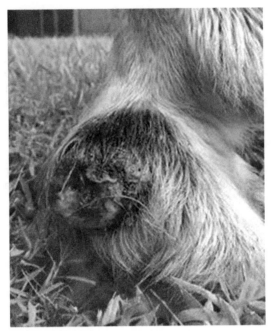

Fig. 2. Fibroblastic mass, with central draining tract. This is a photograph of the infected collateral cartilage seen radiographically in **Fig. 1**.

Kamus and Christine Theoret's article, "Choosing the Best Approach to Wound Management and Closure," in this issue).

Skin Grafting

Skin grafting is a surgical procedure that can be used for nonhealing wounds that are difficult to close due to location, size, or quality of underlying wound tissues. There are several grafting options, some requiring minimal experience and equipment.[23–25]

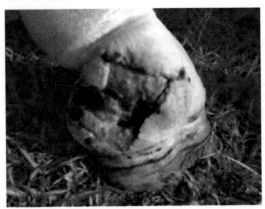

Fig. 3. Skin defect after debulking of the mass and removal of the infected collateral cartilage seen in **Fig. 2**.

Skin graft categories
The 2 main categories of skin grafts include pedicle grafts and free skin grafts.

Pedicle grafts Pedicle grafts are full-thickness skin grafts that are transposed from the donor to the graft site, while still connected to a vascular pedicle. Due to the inelasticity of equine skin, these grafts are rarely used or successful for equine patients.

Free skin grafts Free skin grafts are completely removed from their blood supply and are more typically used for equine patients. Free skin grafts can be further classified based on the source of the graft and the thickness of the graft.

   Source of free skin graft Autografts are free skin grafts acquired from one site and grafted onto a different site of the same horse.
   Autografts have the advantage of lacking a detrimental immune response to the graft as well as being readily available.
   Allografts are free skin grafts acquired from a donor of the same species (different horse).
   Xenografts are free skin grafts acquired from a donor of a different species. Allografts and xenografts can both be useful as biological bandages; however, both result in an immune response that ultimately leads to graft rejection.[26,27]

   Thickness of the free skin graft Full-thickness skin grafts contain epidermis and the entire dermis, whereas split-thickness grafts contain epidermis and some portion of the dermis.
   Full-thickness skin grafts have the advantages of being collected with local anesthesia, providing a more cosmetic appearance, tending to be more durable, and not requiring specialized equipment to obtain. The main disadvantage of full-thickness skin grafts is they are limited to smaller wounds due to lack of redundant skin for a donor site in the horse.
   Split-thickness skin grafts have the advantage of being able to cover larger wounds and likely have an increased acceptance rate compared with full-thickness grafts. The disadvantages of split-thickness include the need for specialized equipment, the need for general anesthesia to obtain the graft due to the discomfort it causes, and poorer cosmetics of both the donor and graft site.[23,24]

Graft acceptance
There are 2 main requirements of a recipient bed to accept a skin graft:

1. Vascularity: free skin grafts lack an active blood supply; therefore, they acquire nutrient supply from the underlying wound bed. Bone that lacks periosteum, tendon that lacks paratenon, and cartilage that lacks perichondrium cannot support skin grafts.[28–31]
2. Freedom from infection and devitalized tissue: infection is the most common cause of skin graft failure and devitalized tissue harbors bacteria and proteolytic enzymes, having a negative impact on graft survival.[28–31]

Physiology of graft acceptance Grafted skin is initially adhered to the wound bed by fibrin from the wound that adheres to the exposed collagen of the graft.[28,32,33] The graft is initially nourished by passive flow via capillary action of plasma from the wound bed through the exposed lumen of blood vessels within the graft. This process is known as plasmatic imbibition.[28,34,35] This source of nutrition lasts for approximately 48 hours. Due to a lack of direct blood supply, the grafts become edematous. After 48 hours, capillaries from the wound bed begin to anastomose with the capillaries from the graft, a process known as inosculation. Over the next 4 days to 5 days, neovascularization and revascularization of the grafts progress, with lymphatic circulation occurring at approximately day 7. At this time, edema begins to resolve.[35] The epidermis becomes hyperplastic during the 2 weeks after grafting. This epidermis can become necrotic and slough, leaving behind a pale dermis.[31] This dermis re-epithelializes from migration of epithelial cells from dermal adnexa. Pigmentation occurs at approximately 4 weeks. Hair can begin to grow at approximately 4 weeks to 6 weeks. Reinnervation, although often incomplete, occurs 7 weeks to 9 weeks after grafting.[29,36] Often, split-thickness grafts appear flaky for several months until eccrine glands regenerate, if they regenerate at all.

Wound preparation It is essential to ensure adequate vascularity to the wound bed and that the wound is free of infection and necrotic material. Fresh granulation tissue accepts a graft better, so débridement of granulation tissue below the skin margin 24 hours to 48 hours prior to grafting is recommended. This débridement encourages capillary sprouting.[37] After débridement, topical antimicrobials can be applied to the wound bed to help keep the bacterial burden low, prior to grafting.

Donor site preparation Donor site preparation depends on the type of grafting being performed. The donor site selected should be in an inconspicuous area due to the possibility of residual defect. In addition, the hair should be removed (clipped, shaved, or chemical depilatory) with attention paid to direction of the hair growth and the skin aseptically prepared. It is essential to ensure the detergent and alcohol are removed by rinsing with sterile physiologic saline. This can help prevent detrimental effects to the grafts.[38]

Recipient site preparation Immediately prior to grafting, the hair surrounding the recipient bed should be clipped and cleansed with physiologic saline only, because the detergents found in surgical scrub have been found to increase the risk of wound bed infection.[38]

Sheet Grafts

Full-thickness sheet grafts
Full-thickness sheet grafts are typically acquired from the cranial pectoral region due to the relative mobility of this skin. These grafts contain epidermis and full dermis. This type of skin graft can typically be acquired in a standing, sedated horse with local anesthesia. Although studies have conflicting results of the effects of local anesthetics on wound healing, it seems prudent to avoid direct infiltration at the site of donor collection.[39] The graft should be slightly larger than the defect it covers. Once a graft is acquired, it should be stretched with the dermis up, to sharply excise the subcutaneous tissue. Visualization of the hair follicles within the dermis confirms adequate removal of the subcutis. The graft can then be attached to the edges of the recipient bed using sutures or staples. The graft should be placed under slight tension to ensure that graft vessels remain open.

Advantages
- Can be acquired in the standing, sedated horse
- Resists trauma and is more cosmetic than split-thickness or island grafts
- No specialized equipment

Disadvantages
- Graft acceptance is less than split thickness due to greater requirement for nutrients and less exposed vascularity available for inosculation.

- Horses lack redundant skin; therefore, full-thickness sheet grafts are limited to small wound defects (typically 8 cm at its widest point).
- Meshing of a graft can allow for larger area coverage; however, equine skin is often too thick for meshing using commercial meshing instruments.

Split-thickness sheet grafts
Split-thickness sheet grafts contain epidermis and varying amounts of dermis. Split-thickness grafts require specialized equipment to perform (ie, dermatome).

Advantages
- Can be harvested in larger sheets than can full-thickness grafts.
- Graft is accepted better than with full-thickness grafts.

Disadvantages
- Less durable and less cosmetic than full-thickness grafts.
- Requires general anesthesia.
- Requires specialized equipment.

Island Grafts

Island grafts are small pieces of either full-thickness or split-thickness skin that are typically inserted into a granulation bed. The most common forms of island grafting are punch grafts, pinch grafts, and tunnel grafts.

Punch grafts
Punch grafts are full-thickness grafts obtained from the donor site using a skin punch (6–8 mm). The donor site should be in an inconspicuous area due to the potential for mild scarring. These sites include the ventrolateral abdomen, the neck under the mane, or the perineum. The donor site should be prepared as described for sheet grafting and desensitized with local anesthetic. The subcutaneous tissues should be excised from the dermis. The donor sites can be left to heal by second intention; however, closure with a suture or staple likely improves cosmetic outcome. Collecting grafts in a symmetric pattern, approximately 1 cm apart, also improves final appearance. Because the subcutaneous dissection can be tedious, a full-thickness sheet graft can be obtained, as described previously, from the pectoral region, and then individual punches can be acquired from this sheet. The donor grafts should be maintained on saline soaked gauze prior to implantation.

The recipient site should be prepared as described for sheet grafting. Starting at the distal aspect of the recipient site, a skin punch 1 size to 2 sizes smaller than the donor punch should be used to remove a plug of granulation tissue. The depth of the granulation plug removed should correspond with the thickness of the graft to be implanted. The grafts should be spaced approximately 6 mm apart. Adequate hemostasis is needed prior to implanting the grafts. This can be achieved by creating the recipient plugs prior to grafting or by inserting sterile cotton tip applicators into each hole until bleeding decreases. Once bleeding is controlled, the donor grafts should be placed within the hole. Once grafting is complete, the site should be covered with a nonadherent dressing, followed by a pressure bandage.

Advantages
- 60% to 75% of implanted grafts are expected to survive.
- Each graft is independent so, unlike sheet grafts, loss of some of the grafts does not lead to total loss.
- Minimal equipment is needed.

- Can be done with a horse standing
- Can be used in conditions where sheet grafts are more likely to fail (ie, motion)

Disadvantages
- Healing largely results in an epithelialized scar with sparse hair.

Pinch grafts
Pinch grafts are similar to punch grafts, although the thickness of the graft varies, thickest (full thickness) at the center and thinning along the periphery (split thickness). The donor site is selected and prepared as for punch grafts. Collection of the donor graft is achieved by tenting (pinch) the skin with tissue forceps (with care not to crush), suture needle, or hypodermic needle and excising this piece of skin using a scalpel blade (**Fig. 4**). Grafts should be approximately 3 mm in diameter. The grafts can be placed on saline soaked gauze prior to implantation.

The recipient site is prepared similar to the punch graft; however, a pocket is made in the granulation tissue using a no. 15 blade inserted at an acute angle, directed distally or downward. The donor graft is then implanted into the pocket, epithelial side up (**Fig. 5**). Once grafting is complete, the site should be covered with a nonadherent dressing, followed by a pressure bandage.

Advantages
- 50% to 75% of implanted grafts are expected to survive.
- Each graft is independent so, unlike sheet grafts, loss of some of the grafts does not lead to total loss.
- Minimal equipment is needed.
- Can be done with a horse standing
- Can be used in conditions where sheet grafts are more likely to fail (ie, motion)

Disadvantages
- Healing largely results in an epithelialized scar with sparse hair.

Tunnel grafts
Tunnel grafts are narrow (2–3 mm wide) strips of skin of varying thickness implanted into the recipient granulation bed. Therefore, an adequate bed of granulation tissue is needed. The donor site is prepared, as previously described. There are several

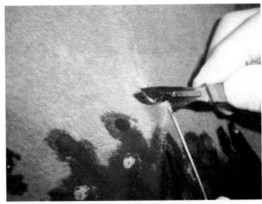

Fig. 4. Pinch graft being obtained from donor site using a hypodermic needle. (*Courtesy of* Richard P. Hackett, DVM, MS, Diplomate, American College of Veterinary Surgeons, Ithaca, NY; with permission.)

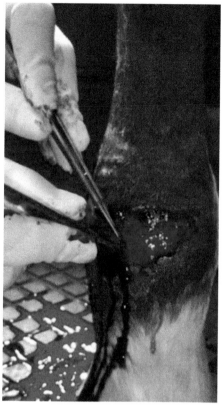

Fig. 5. Pinch graft being inserted into granulation bed. (*Courtesy of* Richard P. Hackett, DVM, MS, Diplomate, American College of Veterinary Surgeons, Ithaca, NY; with permission.)

techniques to acquire the donor skin strips. Subcutaneous wheals (2–3 cm wide and slightly longer than size of the wound being grafted) can be made using local anesthesia at the donor site. The whealed skin is incorporated within the jaws of an intestinal clamp, so that it is protruding above the forceps. The protruding skin is then excised using a scalpel blade along the jaws of the clamp. Alternatively, full-thickness or split-thickness sheets can be obtained as previously described, and these sheets can be cut into 2-mm to 3-mm wide strips.

The recipient site is clipped and prepped as previously described. When tunnel grafting, it can be beneficial for the granulation tissue to be slightly more proud than the wound margin. A long, narrow alligator forceps is tunneled through the granulation bed across the length of the wound at a depth of 5 mm to 6 mm. The donor strip is then grasped and drawn through the tunnel with the epidermis facing the wound surface. The ends of the strip are attached to the wound margin using a suture, staple, or cyanoacrylate. Six days to 10 days after implantation, the roof of the tunnel needs to be excised. This can be accomplished by placing a malleable probe in the tunnel between the roof of the tunnel and the graft and excising over the probe. An alternative is to use a fine wire to saw through the roof of the tunnel. If the graft is implanted at a depth of 1 mm to 1.5 mm, removal of the roof of the tunnel is unnecessary, because it often sloughs within 7 days.[40,41]

Advantages
- 60% to 80% of implanted grafts are expected to survive.
- Can be used in areas of high motion, because the granulation tissue protects the graft from shear forces
- Each graft is independent, so, unlike sheet grafts, loss of some of the grafts does not lead to total loss.
- Minimal equipment is needed
- Can usually be done with a horse standing

Disadvantages
- Healing largely results in an epithelialized scar with sparse hair.
- Removing granulation roof can be difficult and tedious.

Modified meek grafts

Modified Meek grafting is a technique that combines island grafting with split-thickness sheet grafting. After collecting a split-thickness skin sheet (4.2 cm^2), the sheet is passed through a Meek micrograft machine[a], which creates 196 island grafts that are 3 mm^2. The modified Meek grafting technique is useful for large wounds when limited donor skin is available.[42] It has the same advantages of other island grafting techniques but has the disadvantages of split-thickness sheet grafting, such as the need for specialized equipment and for the horse to be anesthetized.

Aftercare of Recipient Site

As described previously, recipient site should be covered with a nonadherent dressing secured with sterile conform gauze, followed by a thick bandage that minimizes motion and has the capability to wick exudate from the grafted site. The initial bandage should not be changed for 4 days to 5 days postgrafting to allow the early fibrinous and vascular attachments to progress with minimal disruption. The nonadherent dressing should be carefully removed by applying pressure parallel to the wound surface, because pulling the dressing perpendicular to the wound surface is more likely to disrupt the graft attachments. If the dressing is firmly adhered to the surface, it can be moistened with sterile saline or left in place until the next bandage change. Topical antimicrobials may be beneficial at keeping local bacterial counts low while the grafts are being accepted.

Tissue Expanders

Another surgical consideration for the nonhealing wound is the use of tissue expanders to allow for reconstructive procedures when limited skin is available. This technique can be particularly useful on distal limb or head wounds. To date, there are few reports of the use of silicone elastomer tissue expanders in the horse. Tissue expanders typically consist of a silicone pouch that can be placed subcutaneously and then gradually inflated with sterile saline via a percutaneous injection into an inflation portal. These pouches are placed adjacent to, but not in contact with, the lesion site. After the implant incision has healed, the expander can be distended every 4 days to 7 days, thereby stretching the overlying skin. Once sufficient skin expansion has occurred, the elastomer is removed and the expanded skin tissue is undermined and used as a skin flap to cover the defect.[7]

---

[a] Humeca- Woodstock, GA.

Tissue expanders can increase the area of skin 2-fold to 3-fold. The epidermis responds to the gradual inflation by an increase in mitotic activity and thus an increase in epidermal tissue. The dermis thins in response to the expansion of the elastomer.[43] Skin flaps made from expanded skin are twice as likely to survive as those created from acutely raised skin.[44]

Tissue expansion in the horse has been associated with complications, such as pain during saline distention, pressure necrosis of the overlying skin, implant failure, wound dehiscence, and premature exposure of the expander requiring its removal before adequate expansion has been achieved.[7] Tissue expanders are expensive and should not be implanted in proximity to neoplastic or septic concerns. Because of these issues and others, the use of tissue expanders has not been widespread in the horse. The authors have had personal communication with a company in the United Kingdom (Oxtex, Witney, UK), that has developed an innovative, uniformly self-expanding hydrogel implant that does not require saline injections into a subcutaneous port. The implant is medical grade and has established safety data in rats, sheep, and horses. Several equine cases have been successfully treated using the novel skin expanders and an article is in preparation. The cases include equine distal limb, head, and rectovaginal reconstructions. The hope is that these novel tissue expanders will increase the surgical options for horses with wounds or masses in locations with limited skin (**Figs. 6–8**).

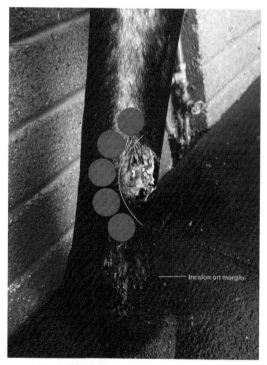

Fig. 6. Chronic nonresponsive inflammatory tissue on the dorsomedial aspect of the left hindlimb. Red circles indicate proposed location of skin expanders; green line is proposed incision. (*Courtesy of* Simon Hennessy MVB MSc Cert AVP [ESO] [ESST] MRCVS DipECVS, Lisadell Equine Hospital, Co. Meath, Ireland; with permission.)

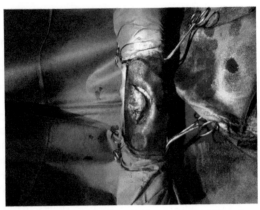

Fig. 7. Intraoperative view showing implanted skin expanders. (*Courtesy of* Simon Hennessy MVB MSc Cert AVP [ESO] [ESST] MRCVS DipECVS, Lisadell Equine Hospital, Co. Meath, Ireland; with permission.)

TREATMENT RESISTANCE/COMPLICATIONS

Resistance to treatment is typically due to failure to resolve the underlying cause of inflammation/infection. Wounds that are in areas of high motion (especially over a joint) can be especially challenging. Some humans receiving skin grafts report that the grafted site can be hyperaesthetic.[29,36] This likely occurs in horses, as demonstrated by the self-mutilation that sometimes occurs once a grafted wound is no longer bandaged.

Wounds that have healed with redundant epithelial scar and minimal adnexa are more prone to being retraumatized.

EVALUATION OF OUTCOME AND LONG-TERM RECOMMENDATIONS

When the underlying complicating issues are addressed and the wound environment is controlled, outcomes for horses with inappropriately healing wounds can be successful.

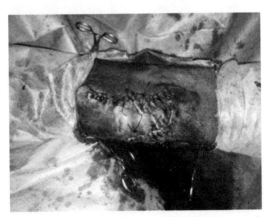

Fig. 8. Intraoperative view of skin closure after removal of tissue expanders and mass. (*Courtesy of* Simon Hennessy MVB MSc Cert AVP [ESO] [ESST] MRCVS DipECVS, Lisadell Equine Hospital, Co. Meath, Ireland; with permission.)

SUMMARY

Nonhealing wounds in horses represent a common challenge to the equine practitioner. The unique healing process of the horse, particularly of the distal limb with poor supportive tissues and a predilection for excess granulation tissue, contributes to this challenge. To successfully resolve a nonhealing wound, it is essential to evaluate the whole patient, identify and resolve any underlying sources of infection or inflammation, and re-establish an ideal environment for wound healing to proceed.

REFERENCES

1. Hendrickson DA. Management of superficial wounds. In: Auer JA, Stick JA, editors. Equine surgery. 4th edition. St Louis (MO): Elsevier; 2012. p. 306–17.
2. Wilmink JM, Stolk PWT, van Weeren PR, et al. Differences in second-intention wound healing between horses and ponies: macroscopical aspects. Equine Vet J 1999;31:53.
3. Wilmink JM, van Weeren PR, Stolk PWT, et al. Differences in second-intention wound healing between horses and ponies: histological aspects. Equine Vet J 1999;31:61.
4. Wilmink JM, van Herten J, van Weeren PR, et al. Study of primary-intention healing and sequester formation in horses compared to ponies. Equine Vet J 2002;34:270.
5. Van Den Boom R, Wilmink JM, O'Kane S, et al. Transforming growth factor-! levels during second intention healing are related to the different course of wound contraction in horses and ponies. Wound Repair Regen 2002;10:188.
6. Borges AF. Elective incisions and scar revision. Boston: Little Brown; 1973.
7. Provost PJ, Bailey JV. Principles of plastic and reconstructive surgery. In: Auer JA, Stick JA, editors. Equine surgery. 4th edition. St Louis (MO): Elsevier; 2012. 272, 271–284.
8. Theoret CL, Wilmink JM. Treatment of exuberant granulation tissue. In: Stashak TS, Theoret CL, editors. Equine wound management. 2nd edition. Ames (IA): Wiley-Blackwell; 2008. p. 445–62.
9. Frank N. Advancing research and providing recommendations for the diagnosis and management of equine endocrine disorders. In: Equine Endocrinology Group. 2017. Available at: https://sites.tufts.edu/equineendogroup/.
10. Dow G. Infection in chronic wounds. In: Krasner DL, Rodeheaver GT, Sibbald RG, editors. Chronic wound care. 3rd edition. Wayne (PA): HMP Communications; 2001. p. 343.
11. Barber SM. Second intention wound healing in the horse: the effect of bandages and topical corticosteroids. Proc Am Assoc Equine Pract 1989;35:107.
12. Blackford JT, Blackford LW, Adair HS. The use of antimicrobial glucocorticosteroid ointment on granulating lower leg wounds in horses. Proc Am Assoc Equine Pract 1991;37:71.
13. Hashimoto I, Nakanishi H, Shono Y, et al. Angiostatic effects of corticosteroid on wound healing on the rabbit ear. J Med Invest 2002;49:61.
14. Stashak TS, Farstvedt E. Update on wound dressings: indications and best use. In: Stashak TS, Theoret CL, editors. Equine wound management. 2nd edition. Ames (IA): Wiley Blackwell; 2008. p. 109–36.
15. Swaim SF, Gilette RL. An update on wound medications and dressings. Comp Cont Educ Prac Vet 1998;20:1133.

16. Ducharme-Desjarlais M, Celesete CJ, Leapult E, et al. Effect of silicone containing dressing on exuberant granulation tissue formation and wound repair in horses. Am J Vet Res 2005;66:1133–9.
17. Carney SA, Cason CG, Gower JP, et al. Cica-Care gel sheeting in the management of hypertrophic scarring. Burns 1994;20:163–7.
18. Gold MH, Foster TD, Adair MA, et al. Prevention of hypertrophic scars and keloids by the prophylactic use of topical silicone gel sheets following a surgical procedure in an office setting. Dermatol Surg 2001;27:641–4.
19. Kischer CW, Shetlar MR, Shetlar CL. Alteration of hypertrophic scars induced by mechanical pressure. Arch Dermatol 1975;111:60–4.
20. Hackett RP. How to prevent and treat exuberant granulation tissue. Proc Am Assoc Equine Pract 2011;57:367–73.
21. Holder TE, Schumacher J, Donnell RL, et al. Effects of hyperbaric oxygen on full-thickness meshed sheet skin grafts applied to fresh and granulating wounds in horses. Am J Vet Res 2008;69(1):144–7.
22. Frykberg RG, Banks J. Challenges in the treatment of chronic wounds. Adv Wound Care 2015;4:560–82.
23. Schumacher J. Skin grafting. In: Auer JA, Stick JA, editors. Equine surgery. 4th edition. St Louis (MO): Elsevier; 2012. p. 285–305.
24. Schumacher J, Wilmink JM. Free skin grafting. In: Stashak TS, Theoret CL, editors. Equine wound management. 2nd edition. Ames (IA): Wiley-Blackwell; 2008. p. 509–42.
25. Hackett RP. How to skin graft in the field. Proc Am Assoc Equine Pract 2011;57:379–84.
26. Bell R. The use of skin grafts. New York: Oxford University Press; 1973.
27. May S. The effects of biological wound dressings on the healing process. Clin Mater 1991;8:243.
28. Argenta LC, Dingman RO. Skin grafting. In: Epstein E, editor. Skin surgery. 6th edition. Philadelphia: Saunders; 1987. p. 129.
29. Flowers RS. Unexpected postoperative problems in skin grafting. Surg Clin North Am 1970;50:439.
30. Rothstein AS. Skin grafting techniques. J Am Podiatry Assoc 1983;73:79.
31. Rudolph R, Fisher JC, Ninnemann JL. Skin grafting. Boston: Little, Brown; 1979.
32. Tavis MJ, Thornton JW, Harney JH, et al. Mechanism of skin graft adherence: Collagen, elastin, and fibrin interactions. Surg Forum 1977;28:522.
33. Teh B. Why do skin grafts fail? Plast Reconstr Surg 1979;63:323.
34. Vistnes LM. Grafting of skin. Surg Clin North Am 1977;57:939.
35. Converse JM, Smahel J, Ballantyne DL, et al. Inosculation of vessels of skin graft and host bed: a fortuitous encounter. Br J Plast Surg 1975;28:274.
36. Fitzgerald MJ, Martin F, Paletta FX. Innervation of skin grafts. Surg Gynecol Obstet 1967;124:808.
37. Smahel J. Free skin transplantation on a prepared bed. Br J Plast Surg 1971;26:129.
38. Edlich RF, Schmolka IR, Prusak MP, et al. The molecular basis for toxicity of surfactants in surgical wounds. J Surg Res 1973;14:277.
39. Waite A, Gilliver SC, Masterson GR, et al. Clinically relevant doses of lidocaine and bupivacaine do not impair cutaneous wound healing in mice. Br J Anaesth 2010;104:768.
40. Bjorck GTK. Tunnel skin grafting in the equine species. Proc Am Assoc Equine Pract 1971;17:313.

41. Lees MJ, Andrews GC, Bailey JV, et al. Tunnel grafting of equine wounds. Comp Cont Educ Prac Vet 1989;11:962.
42. Wilmink JM, van den Boom R, van Weeren PR, et al. The modified Meek technique as a novel method for skin grafting in horses: evaluation of acceptance, wound contraction and closure in chronic wounds. Equine Vet J 2006;38(4): 324–9.
43. Johnson ™, Lowe L, Brown MD, et al. Histology and physiology of tissue expansion. J Dermatol Surg 1993;19:1074.
44. Madison JB. Tissue expansion. Vet Clin North Am Equine Pract 1989;5:633.

Equine Wound Management

Bandages, Casts, and External Support

Randy B. Eggleston, DVM

KEYWORDS

- Bandage • Cast • Cast bandage

KEY POINTS

- Bandages have a substantial impact on wound healing by protecting wounds from further trauma, desiccation, and contamination, and helping reduce hemorrhage and edema.
- Appropriate use of bandages during the debridement stage of wound healing is effective by absorbing and removing surface contamination and debris.
- Rigid casts and splints help to immobilize wounds in areas of high motion, thereby improving wound healing.
- Wounds involving structural support soft tissues (tendons and/or ligaments) benefit greatly from rigid coaptation.

Successful management of equine wounds relies on knowledge of the stages of wound healing, factors that can alter those stages, how healing stages can be manipulated, and adherence to the principles of wound healing. Challenges that complicate wound management include the inability to immobilize and/or confine equine patients, and maintain a clean environment during the critical initial stages of healing. Because of these challenges, the equine practitioner relies heavily on bandaging and external coaptation techniques to successfully treat and manage wounds. The type of bandage used is dictated by the region of the body that is injured. Distal limb wounds are the most conducive to bandaging, whereas wounds to the shoulder and gluteal regions can be difficult to bandage in a traditional manner. Wounds to the head and neck are conducive to bandaging with creative modifications.

BANDAGES

Bandages protect wounds from further trauma, desiccation, and contamination; absorb secretions; aid in debridement; reduce hemorrhage and edema; and reduce motion of the wound. The distal limb is the most common region to bandage due to frequent wounding and the ease of application and maintenance.

The author has nothing to disclose.
Department of Large Animal Medicine, College of Veterinary Medicine, University of Georgia, 2200 College Station Road, Athens, GA 30602, USA
E-mail address: egglesto@uga.edu

Vet Clin Equine 34 (2018) 557–574
https://doi.org/10.1016/j.cveq.2018.07.010
0749-0739/18/© 2018 Elsevier Inc. All rights reserved.

The standard distal limb bandage/wrap is composed of 3 layers: primary, secondary, and tertiary. Each layer serves a specific purpose important to the management of the wound.

Primary Layer

- The primary layer is the most influential layer, as it is in contact with wounded tissues.
- It can be modified in a number of ways to fit the stage of healing and have the most appropriate effect on the wound.
- The primary layer can also be harmful to the wound if not used appropriately.
- The primary layer is classified with respect to the material used, gas and fluid exchange, and the ability of the material to adhere to the wound.[1–3]
  - Synthetic, semisynthetic, or biologic
  - Occlusive, semiocclusive, or nonocclusive
  - Adherent or nonadherent

A synthetic, nonocclusive, or semiocclusive primary layer is the most commonly used for equine wounds. Occlusive dressings are best used in the first 3 to 5 days of healing, as they promote the formation of granulation tissue and delay healing time.[4] An exception to this is the use of synthetic, nonadherent occlusive silicone dressings. Silicone dressings are used extensively in human medicine to reduce scar formation.[5,6] In a study in horses, a silicone-containing dressing outperformed a conventional dressing, resulting in the prevention of exuberant granulation tissue formation and improved tissue quality.[7]

The primary layer can be modified in a number of ways to achieve its desired effects on a particular wound, as it is in direct contact with the wound and plays a major role in the progression of healing (**Fig. 1**). The stage of wound healing dictates the chosen composition of the primary layer. In the initial debridement stage of healing, adherent bandages are indicated where large quantities of necrotic tissue and thick exudate are present. Suggested materials are wide meshed sterile gauze, such as 4 × 4 gauze sponges, which are highly absorbent and allow incorporation of large particles into the mesh of the gauze. Adherent bandages can be further classified as Dry-to-Dry, Wet-to-Dry, or Wet-to-Wet.[1] Dry-to-Dry bandages are used when the wound surface

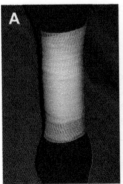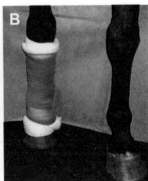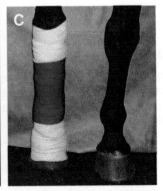

Fig. 1. (*A*) Primary layer composed of a nonadherent dressing held in place by sterile 4-inch Kling gauze. (*B*) Secondary layer composed of 5 layers of sheet cotton held in place with 6-inch brown gauze. (*C*) Tertiary layer composed of 4-inch elastic Vet Wrap. The proximal and distal end of the bandage have been sealed with 4-inch elastic adhesive Elastikon tape.

contains large quantities of loose tissue and low viscous exudate. A layer of dry sterile gauze is placed on the wound with overlying secondary and tertiary layers and left in place until the unwanted material is absorbed and the primary layer is dry. The bandage is then removed, debriding the wound as the gauze is elevated. Removing the primary layer may be painful for a horse and light sedation may be required. Lightly wetting the gauze can help loosen the material and make removal less painful. If additional debridement is necessary, reapplication of a Dry-to-Dry bandage can be done.

Wet-to-Dry bandages are indicated for desiccated wounds that contain dried, viscous, and necrotic material.[2] The moisture of the primary layer helps to soften and loosen the unwanted material and allows it to be absorbed into the mesh of the bandage, and the wound site can be debrided with bandage removal. The primary layer is lightly moistened with sterile saline or an antibacterial solution. If an antibacterial solution is desired, appropriate concentrations should be used (chlorhexidine 0.05%, povidone iodine 0.1%). The bandage is removed once the primary layer has dried. The Wet-to-Dry layer should not be oversaturated; excessive moisture can allow wicking of bacteria through the secondary and tertiary layers. Maceration of the surrounding tissues may also occur.

Wet-to-Wet bandages have little debriding capability. They are indicated for wounds with a large quantity of viscous exudate that lack marked debris and necrotic tissue. Wet-to-Wet bandages are effective at diluting and thinning the exudate, making removal easier. The primary layer is applied wet and is removed wet. A sterile fluid or antimicrobial solution can be used as the wetting agent. The quantity of fluid used should be more than that used for a Wet-to-Dry bandage.

Nonadherent bandages are used when the wound has been satisfactorily debrided. This implies that wound fibroplasia and epithelialization are occurring, and protection of the new granulation tissue and epithelium should be taken into consideration. A nonadherent Telfa (Covidien Ltd. Co., Dublin, Ireland) is a semiocclusive bandage that retains enough moisture to prevent wound dehydration and promote epithelialization. Any excess fluid from the wound also can be absorbed, preventing tissue maceration.[2]

Secondary Layer

The secondary bandage layer is primarily an absorptive layer and adds protection to the wound. This layer absorbs and stores excess drainage of blood, serum, exudate, and necrotic tissue from the wound surface.[3] Secondary layers are usually composed of sheet or roll cotton. The bandage should be of sufficient thickness to adequately absorb and retain the excess fluid and provide a pad over the wound. Three to 4 layers of sheet cotton folded in half, or 2 complete layers of roll cotton, are adequate for most wounds (see **Fig. 1**). This layer should fit snugly, but not so tight that absorption is hindered.

Tertiary Layer

The tertiary layer is the holding layer of the bandage. It is composed of an adhesive tape (Elastikon; Johnson & Johnson, New Brunswick, NJ) or self-bonding material (Vet Wrap [3M Corporation, St. Paul, MN], Co-Flex [Andover Medical, Salisbury, MA]) (see **Fig. 1**). The tertiary layer can be applied with varying pressure. Depending on the type and location of the wound, the tertiary layer can supply some degree of immobilization when applied under pressure. The secondary layer should be of sufficient thickness if the tertiary layer is to be applied under semi-immobilizing pressure. A tightly applied tertiary layer without adequate padding from the secondary layer can cause tissue damage to the skin and underlying tissues (ie, flexor tendons).

The tertiary layer can be applied with moderate pressure without causing danger to the underlying soft tissues, provided 4 to 5 sheets of the sheet cotton or an equivalent material are used. The bandage should be wrapped in the same direction as the primary and secondary layers, otherwise loosening of the bandage will occur. It is important to apply each turn of the wrap with the same amount of pressure. Areas of eccentrically concentrated pressure can cause soft tissue trauma at those areas. A second tertiary layer can be applied if marked edema is present. Six-inch nonelastic brown gauze works well to supply an even distribution of pressure throughout the wrap. Elastikon can be applied to the top and bottom of the bandage to eliminate further contamination with bedding material.

SPECIFIC BANDAGES
Stack Bandage (Full-Limb Bandage)

A stack bandage is commonly used for wounds of the upper limb and to address whole-limb edema (**Fig. 2**). A stack bandage is simply a bandage stacked proximally

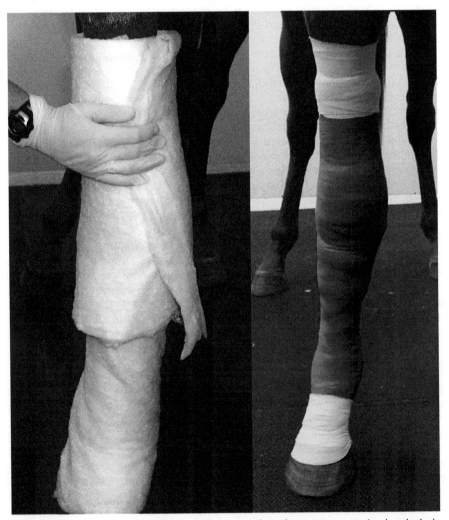

Fig. 2. Stack bandage is indicated for treating wounds to the carpus or proximal and whole-limb swelling.

on top of a distal limb bandage. The distal portion of the bandage helps to maintain the upper portion of the bandage in place. Because of the narrowing distal anatomy of the front limb, maintaining an upper limb bandage can be difficult. A tightly placed upper limb bandage can also induce edema formation in the distal limb. Applying a stack bandage is an effective alternative. Stack wraps also supply padding to the limb when rigid splints are used.

Carpal Bandage

Bandaging wounds of the carpus can be difficult. Use of a stack bandage is one method. Using an adhesive elastic bandage for the tertiary layer is another method. The primary and secondary layers can be applied in similar fashion to a distal limb bandage. The tertiary layer is started well proximal to the secondary layer to achieve adequate anchor to the haired skin of the antebrachium with the adhesive bandage. Elastikon is commonly used. The elastic adhesive tertiary layer should be loosely applied to the skin, and the desired pressure can be applied throughout the secondary layer. When bandaging the carpus, pressure over the accessory carpal bone is a concern. A releasing cut through the tight bandage layers over the accessory carpal bone will relieve the pressure and aid in preventing pressure sores at the site (**Fig. 3**).

Tarsal Bandage

The tarsus also can be a challenge to bandage. Bandage slippage is usually not a problem because of the angle of the hock. Constriction at the point of the common calcaneal tendon and pressure concentration at the point of the hock (calcaneus) are potential problems. Application of a tarsal bandage is similar to a distal limb bandage. When applying the secondary layer, the bandage material should stay aligned with the distal tibia. The material should be pulled taught, pressed flat, and folded evenly over the medial aspect of the tarsus. This will create a smooth, non-wrinkled bandage (**Fig. 4**). The tertiary layer can be applied in a figure of 8 pattern around the point of the hock to reduce pressure over the calcaneus. If complete

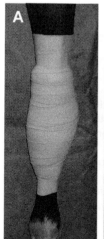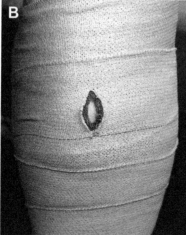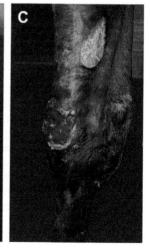

Fig. 3. Carpal bandage. (*A*) An adhesive tertiary layer can help secure to the carpus and prevent slippage. (*B*) Releasing incision over the accessory carpal bone helps to relieve focal pressure over the bone. (*C*) Pressure sore over the accessory carpal bone due to an improperly placed carpal bandage.

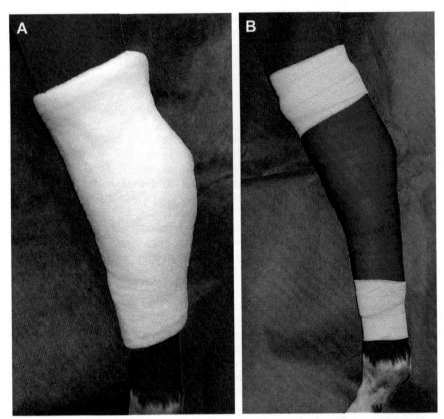

Fig. 4. Tarsal bandage. (*A*) Sheet colon is unrolled in alignment with the tibia. The excess material plantar to the tarsus is placed under light tension and folded over the medial side, forming a smooth secondary layer. (*B*) Completed tarsal bandage. The proximal and distal aspect of the bandage is sealed with Elastikon adhesive tape. The Elastikon also helps prevent slippage.

coverage is desired, a pressure-releasing cut should be made into the bandage over the point of the hock.

CASTS AND SPLINTS

Rigid casts or splints are very useful for management of distal limb wounds when complete or limited immobilization is required. Rigid immobilization is indicated for wounds located in high range of movement regions or when the original wound compromises supporting tissues, such as tendons and ligaments.[8–11] Foot or phalangeal casts are very effective for acute and chronic heel bulb lacerations, hoof wall avulsions, and coronary band trauma.[12,13] Casts also can be applied over sheet grafts to help stabilize the graft and reduce shear forces. Casts applied for wound management are constructed and applied similar to rigid casts used for fracture stabilization (**Table 1**).

Casts can be modified to accommodate the wound management plan. Extensive wounds that involve synovial structures, supporting tendon and/or ligaments, or very exudative wounds requiring frequent bandage changes and wound debridement can be stabilized with a cast bandage. A cast bandage is a combination of a standard 3-layer bandage with an overlying rigid cast.

Table 1
Materials required to construct a standard half-limb cast

Material/Manufacture	Available Splint	Advantages/Disadvantages
Polyvinyl Chloride (PVC) pipe		Inexpensive, readily available, customizable, limited applications.
Fiberglass casting tape		Unlimited constructs, Customizable to multiple applications, single application.
VIP (Veterinary Inclusive Prosthetics/Orthotics)	Prefabricated and custom orthopedic bracing (**Fig. 11**)	Custom fit, expensive
Dynasplint Systems Inc.	Prefabricated and custom orthopedic bracing	Custom fit, expensive
Kimzey Welding Works	Kimzey Leg Saver Splints	Prefabricated, emergency applications, short-term immobilization of wounds, one size for multiple applications.
Red Boot	Equine Limb Saver	Prefabricated, emergency applications, short-term immobilization of wounds, one size for multiple applications.

Similar product was found to be far superior to casting alone. The author uses the above product extensively and finds it to reduce cast sores and improve cast fit.

From Bramlage LR, Embertson RM, Libbey CJ. Resin impregnated foam as a cast liner on the distal equine limb. Proc Am Assoc Equine Pract 1991;37:481–5; with permission.

Distal limb and phalangeal casts for the front limb can be placed with a horse standing or under general anesthesia. Although possible, application of a distal hind limb cast on a standing horse is difficult and may be more safely done under general anesthesia.[14]

Distal Limb Cast Application

Refer to articles by Elce[3] and Auer[14] for more detailed description of cast application.

- Prepare the wound. Place a sterile wound dressing over the wound and hold it in place with cast padding or Kling gauze (Johnson & Johnson). The primary layer should be low mass, as to not result in excessive compression and later cause cast loosening. Use a double layer of stockinet, covering the entire foot and extending above the carpus or tarsus. The stockinet should be snug on the limb to prevent wrinkling beneath the cast.
- Cut a 2-inch to 4-inch-wide strip of casting felt. Cut it to length so it will fit snugly, but completely, around the proximal metacarpus/metatarsus, approximately 2 to 4 cm below the level of the carpometacarpal/tarsometatarsal joint. Secure the ends with 1-inch or 2-inch-white medical tape.
- Drill two 4-mm to 5-mm holes through the hoof wall at the toe and place a 12-inch to 24-inch length of wire through the holes and twist the free ends. This will allow an assistant to secure the limb in a stable position and place the fetlock at the desired angle. If being performed in a standing horse, the limb should be held

by an assistant at the level of the distal radius, allowing the distal limb to hang freely out of weight bearing. A second assistant can then apply tension to the toe wire. In a standing horse, it is very important (once cast application is started) that there is no movement in the limb. Limb movement can create wrinkles in the cast and lead to pressure sores. If unable to off-weight the limb, the cast can be applied in the weight-bearing position, similar to applying the foot cast (see later in this article). It is important that the horse remain standing square and not shifting any weight during application, as this will cause potential complications in the fetlock region.

- (Optional step) Apply a layer of support foam starting at the distal margin of the casting felt; spiraling down the leg, overlapping 50% so there is an even layer throughout. The support foam can be stopped just below the coronary band. This material can be applied under firm tension to prevent wrinkling. A no longer available original product was a resin-impregnated polyurethane foam that was found to be far superior to casting alone.[15] That product has been replaced with a dry polyurethane foam with an adhesive backing, which allows for self-adhered secure application (3M Reston Self-Adhering Foam; 3M Corporation).
- For a half-limb (distal limb) cast, 6 to 7 rolls of 4-inch casting tape are required.
  - Submerse each individual roll in warm water for 10 to 15 seconds. Gently squeeze the tape 3 to 4 times while submersed.
  - Before application, gently ring out excess moisture, leaving the tape moderately wet.
  - Initiate application 1 cm below the top edge of the casting felt. Apply first 2 to 3 wraps directly on top of one another.
  - Spiral the material down the leg, overlapping each wrap by 50%. Timely application is important to prevent premature curing of the material. Most fiberglass casting tapes have a weight-bearing cure time of 20 to 30 minutes. Apply under gentle tension, as not to cause excessive pressure under the cast. Avoid wrinkling or focal finger pressure that may result in pressure points.
  - Initiate second roll 10 to 15 cm proximal to the termination of the first roll. Continue distally to include the foot. Smooth application through the fetlock, pastern, and foot can be difficult. Reversing the direction of application can help. Gently fold the tape over to form the desired direction of application. Once the foot is incorporated, application can continue proximally.
  - Initiate the third roll in similar fashion to the first roll.
  - Following completion of the third roll, fold down excess stockinet evenly, forming a smooth fabric cuff.
  - Continue applying casting tape until you have applied the appropriate 6 to 7 rolls.
- Depending on the desired fetlock angle, the foot may not stand flat to the ground. To prevent undue pressure at the proximal dorsal aspect of the cast, and to broaden the weight-bearing surface, a single roll of 3-inch casting tape can be conformed to the heel region of the cast to form a heel wedge. Secure the wedge onto the cast with a final roll of casting tape.
- Once the cast is hardened, a 2-part acrylic (Technovit; Jorgensen Laboratories, Inc., Loveland, CO) is applied to the bottom of the cast to prevent wearing. Mix approximately 8 oz powder with the appropriate volume of solvent to make a thick paste. Pour the mixture onto a 12 ×12-inch piece of plastic and apply to the bottom of the cast and secure to the foot with white tape. Using this method allows forming the acrylic without direct contact while it sets.

- Apply 2 to 3 loose wraps of Elastikon at the proximal aspect of the cast extending onto the skin. This "seals" the cast from bedding and other debris that might cause tissue irritation.
- Once the cast is set, the author will stand the horse on a flat, even surface and check the fit of the cast. Ideally, the limb should be centered in the cast with minimal pressure throughout the circumference of the cast. It is common to have pressure along the dorsal rim of the cast. Using an electric hand grinder or a Farrier's rasp, material can be removed from the bottom of the cast at the toe region. If ample material is not available to remove, the heel can be built up with additional Technovit. Scoring the existing Technovit with the grinder will improve binding of any new material.

Cast Bandage

A cast bandage is an excellent treatment choice for wounds that would benefit from rigid immobilization but require frequent treatment. A standard 3-layer bandage is first placed on the distal limb. One additional sheet of cotton should be added to the initial bandage. Reapplication of a bivalved cast can be difficult if the desired number of cotton sheets is used for the initial construction of the cast bandage. A standard cast is applied over this bandage. Twenty-four to 48 hours after cast material application, the cast can be cut at the medial and lateral aspects, leaving the solar portion intact. This forms a bivalved splint that can be removed for treatment of the wound. When removing the 2-halves of the cast, the front and back should be gently separated. This will cause the cast to break and hinge at the weight-bearing aspect of the foot. The cast can then be removed distally while the limb is held off the ground. After treatment of the wound, the cast can be carefully replaced on the limb, closed, and secured with a continuous layer of 2-inch medical tape (**Fig. 5**).

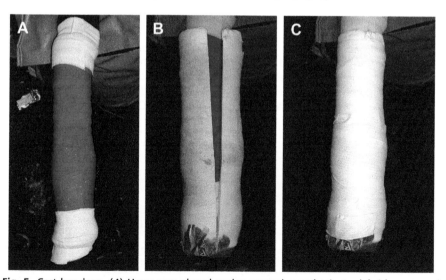

Fig. 5. Cast bandage. (*A*) Horse was placed under general anesthesia to debride a wound involving the metacarpophalangeal joint. Standard 3-layer distal limb bandage has been placed. (*B*) Standard distal limb fiberglass cast was placed over the bandage and allowed to set. Using a cast saw, the cast was cut at 3:00 and 9:00 position. This will allow the cast to act as a bivalve and be removed for later treatment of the wound. (*C*) Completed cast bandage. The cast has been compressed and secured with 2-inch white tape.

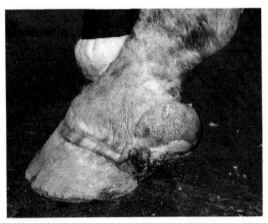

Fig. 6. EGT as the result of an inappropriately treated heel bulb laceration.

Foot Cast

Wounds of the pastern, heel bulb, and hoof wall are common injuries in the horse. These wounds present a particular challenge to wound management.[12,16,17] Suture closure and maintaining closure of an acute heel bulb laceration is difficult due to location and skin tension. If left to heal by second intention, the formation of exuberant granulation tissue is common and further complicates management (**Fig. 6**). Application of a mid-pastern foot cast is a very effective method of stabilization and treatment of these injuries.[8,12]

An acute wound that is not conducive to primary closure can be managed for 7 to 10 days under a bandage,[12] which can allow time for debridement and infiltration of healthy granulation tissue. Once covered with granulation tissue, a foot cast can be applied (**Fig. 7**). An alternative consideration is acute placement of a foot cast once synovial penetration has been ruled out. This can substantially control granulation tissue formation. If communication with a synovial structure is identified, the wound should continue to be managed with a replaceable bandage. Appropriate therapy should be instituted and continued until it can be confirmed that synovial communication no longer exists[18] (see Elsa K. Ludwig and Philip D. van Harreveld's article, "Equine Wounds Over Synovial Structures," in this issue).

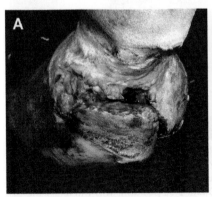
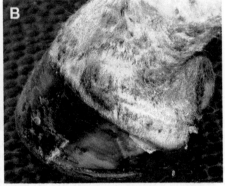

Fig. 7. Severe heel bulb laceration. (*A*) The wound was treated as an open wound and debrided for 7 to 10 days. (*B*) The same wound as in (*A*) after 14 days in a foot cast.

Exuberant granulation tissue (EGT) is often present with chronic distal limb wounds and impedes tissue apposition and normal healing (see **Fig. 6**). The wound should be assessed and debrided of EGT. The foot can then be placed in a well-padded absorptive bandage for hemostasis. A foot cast can be applied 12 to 24 hours later.

A foot cast is applied similarly to a half-limb cast. Depending on the clinician's preference and the temperament of the horse, the cast can be applied with a horse standing or under general anesthesia.[3,8,18]

- Light sedation is recommended to help prevent movement of the affected limb.
- A nonadherent primary layer is applied and lightly covered. No additional bandage is necessary.
- A double layer of stockinet, extending up to the fetlock joint is applied.
- A 1.5 to 2.0-inch strip of casting felt, around the proximal pastern, is secured with a short strip of 1 to 2-inch white tape. A piece of casting felt can also be placed over the heel bulbs to reduce the risk of pressure sore formation. For added protection, a layer of 3M Reston Self-Adhering Foam (3M Corporation) can be applied (**Fig. 8**).
- When applying a cast in a standing horse, it is important to have the distal limb in a natural position and to incorporate a portion of the solar surface of the foot when applying the first 1 to 2 rolls of casting tape. To incorporate the sole, the horse can be stood on a flat board with the palmar/plantar one-half to one-third of the foot overhanging the edge of the board. The board should be of ample height to allow placement of casting tape between the foot and the ground.

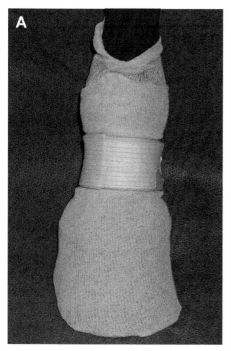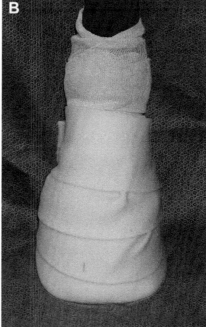

Fig. 8. Foot cast application. (*A*) A double layer of stockinet is applied over the foot extending above the fetlock. A strip of casting felt is secured around the proximal pastern. (*B*) 3M support foam is applied to the pastern and foot (the depicted yellow resin-impregnated foam has been replaced by a dry self-adhesive foam).

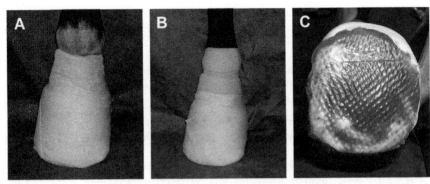

Fig. 9. Foot cast application. (*A*) Two rolls of 4-inch casting tape have been applied to the foot and the excess stockinet has been folded over the proximal rim of the cast. (*B*) The last roll of casting tape had been applied and the cast is complete. The top of the cast has been sealed with 4-inch Elastikon. (*C*) Technovit acrylic has been applied to the bottom of the cast to bolster the wear of the cast.

Standing the opposite foot on a board of equal height will help keep the limbs square.[18] An alternative method is to stand the horse on a wood block that is slightly smaller than the foot. This will allow the entire rim of the hoof and heels to be incorporated in the initial casting.

- Two roles of 3-inch to 4-inch fiberglass cast material should be applied, starting at the proximal pastern spiraling distally, incorporating as much of the solar surface and heel bulbs as possible. The cast should cover the entire foot and extend to the proximal pastern. When the cast is firm to a point that it will not flex, the limb can be picked up and held by an assistant and the residual stockinet folded over the top rim of the cast and the third roll of casting tape applied to incorporate the remainder of the foot (**Fig. 9**).
- To reduce wear of the cast, a layer of Technovit can be applied to the weight-bearing surface of the cast. Elastikon can be placed around the proximal cast to prevent debris from entering the cast (see **Fig. 9**).
- The cast can be left in place for 2 to 4 weeks, which allows for controlled wound healing.
- The rules for cast failure do not necessarily apply to this type of application. The foot cast may become soiled and malodorous with exudative strike through due to the underlying wound. As long as there is no lameness associated with the cast, it should remain in place for the duration of treatment.

Complications

Generally, casts that are applied for the purpose of wound management do not need to be worn longer than 10 to 14 days.[3] Wounds involving tendons and ligaments often require longer coaptation. The most common cast-associated complication is skin injury, or decubital cast sores. Other reported complications include fracture of the cast, superficial digital flexor tendon injury, and long-bone fractures. The incidence of cast sores in the literature is reported to be 45% to 81%.[19–22] One study reported only an 11% incidence of partial-thickness cast sores, but those horses were in casts for less than 15 days.[22]

The most common locations for cast sores are the palmar/plantar aspects of the fetlock and the top of the cast.[19] It is imperative that cast limbs be carefully evaluated multiple times a day, both visually and with palpation of the entire cast. The top of the cast should be evaluated for signs of skin abrasions, moisture, and swelling proximal to the cast. Treatment of visible cast sores includes adjustment of the cast as described earlier, and topical therapy, including a nonadherent dressing with local antimicrobial therapy.

Cast sores located within the confines of a cast can be more difficult to identify early. Lameness and a focal increase in temperature at the site of a sore will be the initial clinical signs.[21] A recent study looking at the use of thermography for the early detection of cast sores found the severity of the cast sore was positively associated with an increase in the temperature differences between the coolest portion of the cast and the affected area, and that the optimal cutoff values for the presence of a superficial, partial-thickness, sore was 2.3°C (4.1°F), and for a deep sore was 4.3°C (7.7°F).[21] As a lesion progresses, the warmth of the affected area will increase. A cast will start to discolor at the affected site due to exudate strike through, and depending on the time of the year, flies may congregate on the cast. As the tissue becomes more abraded and productive, exudate coming from the sore can bubble at the surface of the cast (**Fig. 10**).

Splints

Splints, although not as rigid as a fiberglass cast, work very well in the treatment of equine limb wounds. Splints can be used for distal limb immobilization, but a major indication is for immobilization of wounds involving the carpus and tarsus. Full-limb casts can be used for carpal and tarsal wounds, but the inherent increased risk of complications usually makes the use of a splint more appropriate.[3,19]

Splints can be constructed from various materials at the time of treatment, and pre-fabricated splints are commercially available. A number of commercially available distal limb splints are available and work well, but can be expensive and many of them are not "one-size-fits-all." Custom-made braces are also available through a number of orthotic companies (**Fig. 11, Table 2**).

Polyvinyl chloride (PVC) pipe is probably the most widely used material to fabricate splints. Depending on the size of the limb, 6-inch or 8-inch schedule 40 pipe is recommended. The appropriate length is cut and then using a band saw or cast saw the pipe

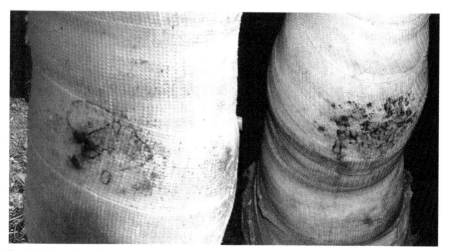

Fig. 10. Examples of cast sores. Note the accumulation of flies at a site of light discoloration of the cast. The image on the right represents a cast sore that has become more productive, resulting in exudate percolating through the cast.

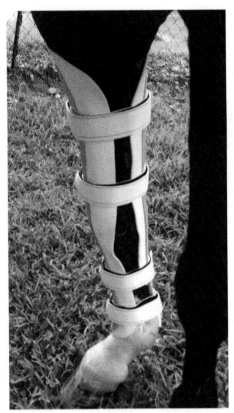

Fig. 11. Example of a commercial custom padded clamshell full-limb splint. The splint is made to conform perfecting to a particular patient and allow access to any underlying wounds.

is cut to form 2 equal halves. Less radius can be used, but rigidity will be decreased as width (circumference) decreases. If molding a splint is required to fit the distal limb, a one-third radius cut will work better and still maintain adequate rigidity. Sharp edges can be rounded with a Farrier's rasp or an electric sander.

For immobilization of the carpus, a splint should extend from the proximal radius to the fetlock joint. Once a wound has been addressed, a well-padded stack wrap should be placed over the entire limb. A splint is fitted to the caudal aspect of the limb and held firmly in place with 2-inch white tape. It is important that the full extent of the splint is securely taped.

For immobilization of the distal limb, a splint should extend from the proximal metacarpus/tarsus down to the ground. To maintain normal conformation of the fetlock and foot, the splint may need modification or extra bandage material. If PVC material is being used, the distal one-fourth to one-third can be heated and molded to match the fetlock angle. Once the material becomes malleable and the appropriate angle is obtained, dipping the splint into cool water will help speed the hardening time of the splint (**Fig. 12**). If circumstances prevent molding the splint, the space palmar/plantar to the pastern and heel bulbs can be filled with a rolled towel or bandage material. This will fill that space between the foot and the splint and keep fetlock angles normal.

Table 2
Examples of available splinting material and manufactured splints

Material/Manufacture	Available Splint	
Polyvinyl chloride (PVC) pipe		$, easily obtained. Can be easily customized. Limited applications.
Fiberglass casting tape		$$, unlimited constructs. Can be molded for multiple applications. Generally single application.
VIP (Veterinary Inclusive Prosthetics/ Orthotics)	Prefabricated and custom orthopedic bracing (see Fig. 11)	$$$
Dynasplint Systems Inc.	Prefabricated and custom orthopedic bracing	$$$
Kimzey Welding Works	Kimzey Leg Saver Splints	$$, Prefabricated brace marketed for emergency break-down injuries. Works well for short-term immobilization for wound management. One size can fit multiple horses.
Red Boot	Equine Limb Saver	$$$

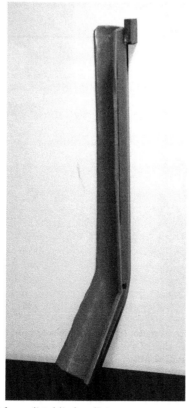

Fig. 12. PVC pipe molded for a distal limb splint.

Fiberglass casting tape also works well for splint fabrication, and has an advantage over PVC material in that it can be molded to the desired region of the limb resulting in a well-fitted custom splint. The disadvantage is the cost of materials.

- Technique-1:
  - Measure the desired length of the splint
  - Using 4-inch or 5-inch tape, wet the material, and on a flat surface quickly fanfold the material to the desired thickness (2–4 rolls). If assistance is available, this step can be performed directly over the limb. The splint can also be constructed dry and submersed before application.
  - Quickly place and conform the malleable material over the limb. Secure the material to the limb with adhesive or self-adhering tape while it cures.
- Technique-2:
  - Apply a standard cast or tube cast bandage as described.
  - Once cured, cut along the medial and lateral aspects, forming 2 halves.
  - Using the desired half of the cast, secure it to the bandaged limb with 2-inch white tape. This technique results in a stronger splint but requires the use of more material.

A recent retrospective evaluated a new design of support brace for distal limb injuries involving partial or complete transection of the superficial digital flexor tendon

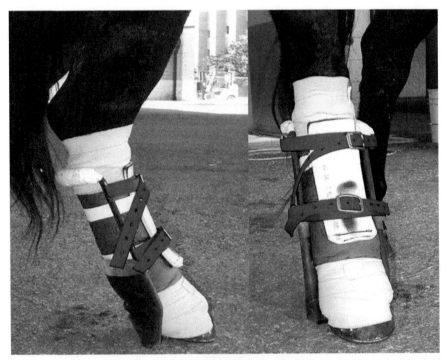

Fig. 13. Fetlock support brace. A metal frame is constructed out of 0.5-inch steel rod, which is attached a preshaped steel shoe. Using additional materials, 4-inch to 6-inch inner tube, PVC pipe, and nylon strapping the affected limb is secured to the brace, resulting in a stable construct that allows for frequent access to the wound for treatment. (*Data from* Whitfield-Cargile C, Babareiner RM, Sustaire D. Use of a fetlock support brace to manage lacerations of equine flexor tendons. Eq Vet Ed 2011;23(1):46–52; and *Courtesy of* Canaan Whitfield, DVM, PhD, College Station, TX; with permission.)

(SDFT) and/or deep digital flexor tendon (DDFT).[23] The brace, once conformed to the limb, is attached to a preshaped and modified steel shoe. Using rubber tubing, PVC, and nylon strapping, the splint supports the fetlock in a stable position and prevents overextension of the distal limb (**Fig. 13**). Of the 15 horses included in the report, 40% had complete transection of the DDFT and SDFT, 26% had complete transection of the SDFT with no damage to the DDFT, and 20% had at least 75% fiber disruption of the DDFT and SDFT. Sixty percent of horses were able to return to previous levels of use and had significantly shorter hospitalization periods (mean 4.2 days). The outcome for horses in this report was similar to previous reports looking at cast immobilization, but the use of the support brace resulted in faster discharge from the hospital, lower overall need for veterinary supervision following discharge, and lower costs to the owner. The brace gives an alternative for those horses that need frequent wound management and have substantial financial constraints.

SUMMARY

Most equine limb wounds benefit from some type of bandaging or coaptation. Bandages play an important role in the overall management of wounds, particularly during the inflammatory and debridement phases. Wounds that are complicated by marked tissue damage, tissue loss, limb instability, and involvement of synovial and supporting soft tissue structures benefit greatly from coaptation to immobilize areas of high motion. Incorporating appropriate bandages and rigid coaptation to the management plan will optimize the rate and quality of wound healing.

REFERENCES

1. Gomez JH, Hanson RR. Use of dressings and bandages in equine wound management. Vet Clin North Am Equine Pract 2005;21:91–104.
2. Stashak TS, Farstvedt E, Othic A. Update on wound dressings: indications and best use. Clin Tech Equine Pract 2004;3:148–63.
3. Elce YA. Bandaging and casting techniques for wound management. In: Theoret CL, Schumacher J, editors. Equine wound management. 3rd edition. Ames (IA): Wiley-Blackwell; 2016. p. 132–55.
4. Howard RD, Stashak TS, Baxter GM. Evaluation of occlusive dressings for management of full-thickness excisional wounds on the distal portion of the limbs of horses. Am J Vet Res 1993;54:2150–4.
5. Carney SA, Cason CG, Gower JP, et al. Cica-Care gel sheeting in the management of hypertrophic scarring. Burns 1994;20:163–7.
6. Gold MH, Foster TD, Adair MA, et al. Prevention of hypertrophic scars and keloids by the prophylactic use of topical silicone gel sheets following a surgical procedure in an office setting. Dermatol Surg 2001;27:641–4.
7. Ducharme-Desjarlais M, Celeste CJ, Lepault E. Effect of a silicon-containing dressing on exuberant granulation tissue formation and wound repair on horses. Am J Vet Res 2005;66:1133–9.
8. Booth TM, Knottenbelt DC. Distal limb casts in equine wound management. Equine Vet Educ 1999;11(5):273–80.
9. O'Sullivan CB. Injuries of the flexor tendons: focus on the superficial digital flexor tendon. Cl Tech Equine Pract 2007;6:189–97.
10. Jordana M, Wilderjans H, Boswell J, et al. Outcome after lacerations of the superficial and deep digital flexor tendons, suspensory ligament and/or distal sesamoidean ligaments in 106 horses. Vet Surg 2011;40:277–83.

11. Tenney WA, Whitcomb MB. Rupture of collateral ligaments in metacarpophalangeal and metatarsophalangeal joints n horses: 17 cases (1999-2005). J Am Vet Med Assoc 2008;233:456–62.

12. Janicek JC, Dabareiner RM, Honnas CM, et al. Heel bulb lacerations in horses: 101 cases (1988-1994). J Am Vet Med Assoc 2005;226:418–23.

13. Celeste CJ, Szöke MO. Management of equine hoof injuries. Vet Clin North Am Equine Pract 2005;21:167–90.

14. Auer AA. Drains, bandages, and external coaptation. In: Auer AA, Stick AA, editors. Equine surgery. 4th edition. St Louis (MO): Elsevier-Saunders; 2012. p. 214–8.

15. Bramlage LR, Embertson RM, Libbey CJ. Resin impregnated foam ass a cast liner on the distal equine limb. Proc Am Assoc Equine Pract 1991;37:481–5.

16. Parks AH. Wounds of the equine foot: principles of healing and treatment. Equine Vet Educ 1997;9(6):317–27.

17. Blackford JT, Latimer FG, Wan PY, et al. Treating pastern and foot lacerations with a phalangeal cast. Proc Am Assoc Equine Pract 1994;40:97–8.

18. Fitzgerald BW, Honnas CM, Plummer AE, et al. How to apply a hindlimb phalangeal cast in the standing patient and minimize complications. Proc Am Assoc Equine Pract 2006;52:631–5.

19. Janicek JC, McClure SR, Lescun TB, et al. Risk factors associated with cast complications in horses: 398 cases (1997–2006). J Am Vet Med Assoc 2013;242:93–8.

20. Lescun TB, Rothenbuhler R, Hawkins JF, et al. A comparison of minimally invasive and open techniques for arthrodesis of the proximal interphalangeal joint in the horse. In: Proceedings of the 16th Annual Scientific Meeting ECVS. Ireland, June 28-30, 2007. p. 163–5.

21. Levet T, Martens A, Devisscher L, et al. Distal limb cast sores in horses: risk factors and early detection using thermography. Equine Vet J 2009;41(1):18–23.

22. Knox PM, Watkins JP. Proximal interphalangeal joint arthrodesis using a combination plate-screw technique in 53 horses (1994-2003). Equine Vet J 2006;38:538–42.

23. Whitfield-Cargile C, Babareiner RM, Sustaire D. Use of a fetlock support brace to manage lacerations of equine flexor tendons. Equine Vet Educ 2011;23(1):46–52.

Equine Wounds over Synovial Structures

Elsa K. Ludwig, DVM, MS, Philip D. van Harreveld, DVM, MS*

KEYWORDS

- Equine • Wound • Synovial • Septic arthritis • Synovitis

KEY POINTS

- Septic synovitis commonly occurs secondary to traumatic wounds that are adjacent to, or communicate with, a synovial structure. Synovial sepsis can be debilitating due to the resulting degenerative changes.
- Treatment goals include rapid resolution of infection, reduction of inflammation, pain management, and the restoration of normal synovial physiologic functions.
- Synovial fluid collection and analysis is the most important diagnostic tool to confirm synovial sepsis.
- A combination of systemic, regional, and/or intrasynovial antibiotics; joint lavage; wound debridement; and analgesic and antiinflammatory medications are often necessary for the treatment of wounds that involve synovial structures.
- Timely diagnosis and treatment of wounds involving synovial structures is critical for obtaining a successful outcome in affected horses.

In adult horses, septic synovitis most commonly occurs secondary to traumatic wounds that are adjacent to, or communicate with, a synovial structure.[1,2] Organic material or bacteria introduced through a wound into a synovial structure can result in inflammation and infection, disrupted homeostasis, and metabolic changes, and these abnormalities can progress to degenerative joint disease, tenosynovitis, or bursitis.[3,4] Synovial sepsis can be a debilitating disorder due to difficulties clearing established infections and the degenerative changes that result from ongoing inflammation.[5,6]

The distal limbs of horses have minimal soft tissue protection, thus wounds in these areas are more likely to have involvement of adjacent synovial structures.[3] Within an affected synovial structure, the degrees of the inflammatory and immunologic responses depend on factors such as the horse's age and immune status, presence of preexisting synovial pathology, virulence and concentration of the microorganism introduced, and duration of infection.[7,8]

Disclosure Statement: The authors have no conflicts of interest to disclose.
Vermont Large Animal Clinic, Equine Hospital, 1054 Lake Road, Milton, VT 05468, USA
* Corresponding author.
E-mail address: vlacvt@gmail.com

Synovial inflammation, fluid changes, fibrin accumulation, organism proliferation, and pain due to established synovial infection require multimodal therapies for successful control and resolution.[2] Prompt diagnosis of a septic synovial structure allows for immediate treatment, improving the prognosis.[9] After treatment of synovial infection, 56% to 81% of horses can return to their original function.[1,10] Goals for successful treatment of infected synovial structures due to wounds include early and accurate recognition of the condition, rapid resolution of pain and inflammation, complete elimination of microorganisms, appropriate healing of the original wound, and a timely return to function.[2,5]

INCIDENCE AND PATHOPHYSIOLOGY OF SYNOVIAL WOUNDS AND INFECTIONS

Hematologic spread or the direct introduction of bacteria or fungi into a synovial structure can result in septic arthritis, tenosynovitis, or bursitis.[11] Penetrating wounds are the most common cause of septic arthritis in adult horses.[1] Synovial structures most commonly affected with infection due to traumatic wounds are the fetlock joint (32.6%), tendon sheaths (21.7%), tarsus (17.4%), coffin joint (13%), navicular bursa (6.5% of synovial structures), carpus (4.3%), stifle joint (2.2%), and pastern joint (2.2%).[1] Contusions or abrasions near synovial structures can result in synovial infection that develops within a few days of injury, because organisms within the infected, surrounding soft tissue can move through the damaged synovium and into the synovial structure.[8] Commensal microorganisms on the horse's skin or within the environment are the bacteria generally involved in synovial infections. *Staphylococcus aureus*, *Pseudomonas spp.*, Enterobacteriaceae, and other staphylococci species are commonly isolated bacteria.[5,12] Other infecting bacteria include *Escherichia coli*, *Salmonella spp.*, *Corynebacterium pseudotuberculosis*, streptococci species, and anaerobic species.[1,11]

The introduction of microorganisms into the synovial membrane or synovial fluid results in an inflammatory reaction, microorganism proliferation and attachment, and the establishment of active infection within the synovial structure.[2,7] Normally, the synovial membrane prevents bacterial proliferation and infection through the phagocytic properties of certain synovial cells and the actions of inflammatory mediators and cytokines produced by synovial cells.[5,7,13] Synovial damage, organism pathogenicity and virulence, and the number of microorganisms inoculated into the synovial structure all contribute to whether the synovial structure's defense mechanisms are overcome and infection is established.[5,7] Within an affected synovial structure, inoculated microorganisms can release extracellular toxins and enzymes, bind to the synovial tissues, and proliferate.[7] The synovium responds to this bacterial colonization by releasing inflammatory mediators, enzymes, and free radicals.[5,7] This can increase vascular permeability, resulting in intrasynovial hemorrhage and extravasation of macrophages, neutrophils, and fibrin into the compartment.[5,11]

Neutrophils kill bacteria by phagocytosis and by releasing enzymes such as oxygen-derived free radicals, cathepsin G, collagenase, elastase, lysozyme, or gelatinase.[7] Free radicals cleave proteoglycans, collagen, and hyaluronic acid, which can lower synovial fluid viscosity, reducing boundary lubrication and biomechanical protection.[7,11,14] Inflammatory mediators activate synoviocytes and chondrocytes, resulting in the production of inflammatory cytokines such as interleukin 1 (IL-1), IL-6, and tumor necrosis factor alpha (TNFα).[11] IL-1 and TNFα increase the production of matrix metalloproteinases (MMP) by activated chondrocytes, synoviocytes, macrophages, fibroblasts, osteoblasts, and endothelial cells.[14,15] The main classes of MMP are stromelysins, gelatinases, and collagenases, which contribute to the breakdown of proteoglycans, collagens, and elastins.[14,15] In addition, MMP presence can cause cartilage degradation, cartilage fibrillation, and chondrocyte necrosis, perpetuating the intrasynovial inflammatory process.[14] Furthermore, the response to infection leads to synovial effusion, increased intrasynovial pressure, reduced blood flow to the synovium, ischemia of subchondral bone and synovial structures, and pain.[5,7]

The extravasation of fibrin from the synovial membrane results in fibrin deposition and free fibrin within the synovial fluid.[5,7] The presence of fibrin can lead to the formation of pannus, which is an intrasynovial fibrinocellular accumulation of tissue, foreign material, and bacteria.[5,7] Organisms within the pannus can be protected from phagocytic white blood cells and antimicrobial agents in the synovial fluid.[11]

If untreated, sepsis can result in substantial synovial structure and cartilage damage.[2] The destruction and loss of proteoglycan and collagen reduces the biomechanical resistance of cartilage, leading to articular cartilage loss and osteoarthritis.[11,14] The resulting synovial changes can prevent a horse from returning to work and may even be severe enough to necessitate euthanasia.

IDENTIFICATION OF WOUNDS OVER SYNOVIAL STRUCTURES
Clinical Signs

When presented with a horse having a wound over a synovial structure, the veterinarian should obtain a patient history and perform a complete physical examination.[2,4] The history will help determine the duration of infection, possible microorganisms involved, and the horse's tetanus prophylaxis status.[2] Because of increased intrasynovial pressure, hypersensitivity of the synovial membrane, and surrounding soft tissue inflammation, horses with septic synovial structures are often very lame (non–weight-bearing lame, American Association of Equine Practitioners grade 5).[5,16] However, if the affected synovial structure is open and draining or if analgesic medications were recently administered, minimal to no lameness may be present.[4,5] In addition, lameness may be less severe if the injury occurred shortly before evaluation.[4,7]

A careful physical examination should evaluate for evidence of trauma or wounds, such as presence of blood or exudate on the skin.[2] Clipping hair may be required to see small puncture wounds, which can quickly seal and are difficult to identify.[2] Vital parameters can vary, with heart rate and respiratory rate ranging from normal to elevated, depending on the level of pain.[4,5] Perisynovial soft tissue heat and swelling, synovial structure effusion, and sensitivity to palpation and manipulation of the synovial structure are clinical findings associated with synovial infection.[5,7] Affected adult horses usually do not have substantial change to their peripheral blood analysis.[5,7] However, the most common complete blood count abnormalities include an elevated white blood cell count, mild neutrophilia, and mild hyperfibrinogenemia.[4,5,7] Horses with infected synovial structures are not consistently febrile or depressed, and therefore, these clinical findings should not rule synovial sepsis in or out.[3,4,17]

Wound Preparation and Exploration

Before exploring a wound with a suspect open septic synovial structure, proper wound preparation is essential. Typically the edges of the wound should be clipped and debris removed. Placement of sterile, water-based lubricating gel in the bed of a wound before clipping can help prevent further contamination, especially in wounds where primary closure is being considered. The wound should be aseptically cleaned with an antiseptic solution and lavaged with sterile saline. Aggressive wound lavage using high volumes of sterile lavage solutions under pressures up to 15 psi can help decrease bacterial numbers and wound contaminants. This can easily be accomplished by using a 35-mL syringe and a 19-gauge needle. After thorough cleaning, exploration of a wound using sterile gloves can be performed. If no obvious communications of the wound with a synovial structure can be identified, distention of a joint or tendon sheath may be required to determine if there is communication. Before distention of a synovial structure, collection of synovial fluid for analysis and culture should be attempted. Care should be taken not to advance needles through infected or compromised periarticular tissue during synoviocentesis. The safest possible approach distant from the wound should be used to minimize the possibility of iatrogenic contamination. Once a needle has been placed into the synovial compartment and a sample obtained, sterile saline or lactated Ringer solution should be infused under pressure to determine if any fluid egresses from the wound (**Fig. 1**). If fluid does not exit through the wound, and intrasynovial pressure builds, the synovial structure is not likely involved. The veterinarian may choose to infuse the suspected compartment with an antibiotic before removing the needle.

Diagnostic Imaging

Diagnostic imaging of a suspected area via radiography, ultrasonography, nuclear scintigraphy, computed tomography (CT), or MRI can aid in determining if a wound involves a synovial structure and if sepsis is established.[2] A complete radiographic

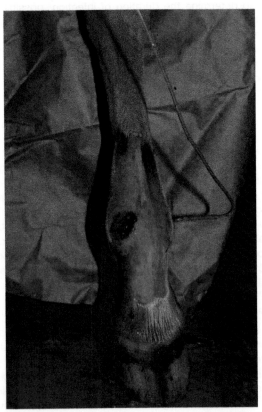

Fig. 1. Sterile saline being infused into fetlock joint to help determine if there is communication with the adjacent wound.

series of an affected joint is warranted for evaluation of bone involvement, such as fractures, physitis, osteomyelitis, osteitis, or osteoarthritis.[5,7] Other than the rare presence of air within a synovial capsule, radiographic signs are most commonly normal in the acute stages after wounding. The presence of bone lysis in association with a septic joint raises the level of concern and will negatively affect prognosis. Contrast radiography, such as fistulograms or the intrasynovial injection of radiographic contrast solution, can be used to determine communication of a wound with a synovial structure or to help reveal cartilage defects (**Fig. 2**).[5,7]

Ultrasonography can be used to evaluate joint, tendon sheath, or bursal effusion, and ultrasound is generally noninvasive.[5,7,18] In addition, ultrasonography can identify inflammation of the synovium, foreign bodies within a synovial compartment or surrounding tissues, and communication between an adjacent wound and a synovial structure.[5,7,18] Ultrasonographic findings in horses affected with synovial sepsis include marked synovial effusion (81% of cases), moderate to severe synovial thickening (69%), presence of intrasynovial fibrin (64%), echogenic synovial fluid (55%), and focal hyperechogenic areas (33%).[18]

Although infrequently used to assess septic synovial structures, nuclear scintigraphy, CT, and MRI can be used to localize infection or inflammation.[2] Although they provide excellent detail of soft tissues and bones, MRI and CT are expensive and may require general anesthesia. These imaging modalities can help determine if lameness is due to chronic synovitis and osteoarthritis, if there is ongoing infection, or if there is a nidus of infection.[19]

Synovial Fluid Collection and Analysis

Synovial fluid collection and analysis is the most important diagnostic tool to confirm synovial sepsis.[2,4] By providing information regarding the severity of inflammation within the synovial structure, synovial fluid analysis helps to distinguish between septic synovitis, nonseptic synovitis, and normal structures.[17,20] The large amount of

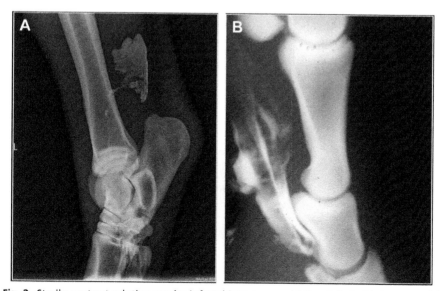

Fig. 2. Sterile contrast solution can be infused into a wound (*A*) or injected into a synovial structure (*B*) to determine communication between a wound and a synovial structure.

variability in clinical symptoms and changes in synovial fluid parameters can make it difficult to properly diagnose septic synovitis.[2] Normal synovial fluid is transparent to pale yellow in color, the fluid's total nucleated cell count (TNCC) is very low (less than 500 cells/μL), and the total protein (TP) concentration is less than 2.0 g/dL.[13,15,20] Normal cellular composition is 90% mononuclear cells, and the remaining 10% of cells are usually neutrophils.[20,21] Normal synovial fluid is viscous due to its hyaluronic acid content, and it does not clot because it does not contain clotting factors or fibrinogen.[13,15,20] Synovial fluid is generally considered to be septic when it has a TP greater than 4.0 g/dL, a TNCC greater than 30,000 cells/μL, and a cellularity greater than 80% neutrophils.[20,22,23]

Synovial fluid collection should be aseptically performed to prevent the introduction of microorganisms or debris during synoviocentesis.[20] Following collection of synovial fluid, the needle can remain within the synovial structure for distension with sterile fluids (see wound exploration, discussed earlier). Collected synovial fluid should be used for cytologic evaluation, culture and sensitivity, and other analyses.[2] A routine synovial fluid analysis includes evaluation of gross appearance (color, turbidity, viscosity), TP concentration, TNCC, and fluid cytology.[20]

Synovial fluid may contain blood from iatrogenic trauma after synoviocentesis; however the entire sample is usually not bloody in this situation.[20] In contrast, hemorrhage from inflamed synovium results in a uniformly bloody synovial fluid sample.[20] Septic synovial fluid may be serosanguinous in color, cloudy, turbid, and nonviscous (**Fig. 3**).[17,20] As a result of synovial inflammation, increased fluid cellularity causes the fluid to seem turbid, and the enzymatic breakdown of hyaluronic acid reduces

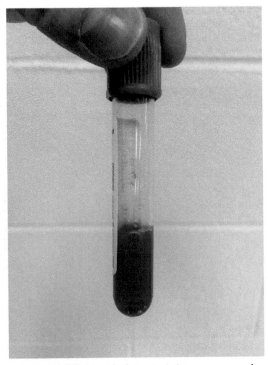

Fig. 3. Sample of septic synovial fluid with characteristic appearance abnormalities (serosanguinous in color, cloudy, and turbid).

the fluid's viscosity.[20] Synovial inflammation damages synovial vessels, resulting in protein leaking from these vessels and increasing the synovial fluid TP concentration.[7,20] The increase in TP concentration is related to the duration and severity of the disease process, with septic synovial fluid usually having TP concentrations greater than 4.0 g/dL, whereas nonseptic synovial inflammation results in lower concentrations.[20,23]

Diagnosis of sepsis should not be based solely on TP concentrations, because concentrations of less than 2.5 g/dL have been reported in cases with positive synovial fluid bacterial cultures.[24] Changes in synovial fluid TNCC can take 12 to 24 hours after inoculation, and a TNCC greater than 30,000 cells/μL suggest synovial sepsis.[7,11,23] The predominant cell type in septic synovial fluid is the neutrophil; neutrophil counts greater than 80% of the nucleated cells are common, and these neutrophils are often normal in appearance or rarely have degenerative changes.[22]

A positive bacterial culture from synovial fluid is often considered to be the gold standard for the diagnosis of septic arthritis. In addition, bacterial culture determines the present microorganisms and sensitivity and susceptibility testing aids in the selection of an appropriate antimicrobial drug.[11] However, the isolation and growth of synovial fluid bacteria can be challenging. Bacteria can be hidden in the pannus or synovial membrane, and cultures from infected joints are negative in almost 50% of clinical cases.[20,24,25] One study showed that when synovial fluid samples had no bacterial growth on initial culture, the reculture of samples that were incubated in blood culture medium for 24 hours resulted in a positive bacterial culture for all samples.[26] A synovial fluid sample should be collected for bacterial culture and sensitivity before the administration of antibiotics.[2] As bacterial culture can take several days to provide results, a Gram stain can be performed on a synovial fluid sample immediately following collection. Although a Gram stain of synovial fluid has a low rate of detection for bacteria, it is positive for microorganisms in about 25% of clinical cases. If bacteria are identified earlier, appropriate antimicrobial selections can procede.[1,20]

Additional Diagnostics

Horses with synovial inflammation (synovitis) can have clinical signs that are very similar to horses with septic synovitis.[17] Nonseptic synovitis due to synovial trauma can result in synovial fluid TNCC, TP concentrations, and cytologic findings equivalent to classic septic synovial fluid parameters.[17,20] Alternatively, horses early in the septic disease process, infection with an organism of low virulence, or nonseptic inflammation can result in synovial fluid TNCC less than 30,000 cells/μL.[20] Therefore, the combination of clinical signs, physical examination findings, wound exploration, diagnostic imaging, and a complete synovial fluid analysis is essential for an accurate diagnosis. The use of additional diagnostics may be warranted to help confirm a diagnosis of synovial sepsis. Commonly used additional diagnostic exercises include the measurement of synovial fluid pH, lactate concentration, glucose concentration, MMP activity, and the activity of myeloperoxidase.[2,20,27,28] In addition, serum amyloid A (SAA) concentration can be a useful aid in the diagnosis of synovial sepsis.[17]

SAA is an acute phase protein that increases in response to inflammation or infection.[2,17,29] Generally, systemic SAA markedly increases in response to bacterial or viral infections, whereas local inflammation usually results in mild to moderate concentration increases.[2,17,30,31] SAA concentrations increase quickly in response to infection and inflammation, and its short half-life makes it a good diagnostic test for monitoring disease progression and response to treatment.[17,31,32] The liver mainly produces SAA isoforms, but specific isoforms are produced locally in certain tissues, including within synovial structures.[2,17,29,31,33] Both serum and synovial fluid SAA concentrations can increase with synovitis and septic arthritis, with the most substantial SAA elevations occurring with septic arthritis.[17,29] In addition, serum SAA concentrations begin to increase 12 hours before synovial fluid SAA concentrations, making it an earlier marker for sepsis.[17] Serum SAA quantification can easily be performed via simple blood collection and the use of a handheld SAA assay (Epona Biotech Limited, Ireland) and can be used as a convenient diagnostic and monitoring modality.[2,17]

The combination of clinical signs, examination findings, and diagnostic results help determine whether a wound involves a synovial structure and whether the synovial structure is infected. If the cumulative diagnostic results suggest sepsis, abrupt treatment is warranted.[4,8] If in doubt, it is always appropriate to assume synovial sepsis is present until proven otherwise.

TREATMENT OF WOUNDS AND SEPTIC SYNOVIAL STRUCTURES

After diagnosis that a wound involves a synovial structure, immediate and aggressive treatment should be implemented to manage both the wound and the synovial structure. The goals of treatment include rapid resolution of infection, reduction of inflammation, pain management, and the restoration of normal synovial physiologic functions.[2,8,34] A combination of systemic, regional, and/or intrasynovial antibiotics; joint lavage; wound debridement; and analgesic and antiinflammatory medications are often necessary for the treatment of wounds that involve synovial structures.

Antimicrobial Therapy

Broad-spectrum antibiotics should be administered following the collection of synovial fluid and continued until otherwise indicated by the synovial fluid bacterial culture and sensitivity results.[5] Most often, a combination of local, regional, and systemic antibiotics are indicated for treatment of synovial sepsis. Systemic antibiotics can be administered orally, intramuscularly, or intravenously.[2] Intravenous antimicrobials are often advised in the acute stages after injury, and oral antibiotics can be administered when the prolonged presence of antibiotics is required after the septic process seems to be resolving (**Tables 1** and **2**).

If no improvement in clinical signs is noted after 72 hours of treatment, diagnostic efforts should be repeated and treatment altered accordingly.[5,8] Antibiotic administration should be continued for 2 to 4 weeks following the resolution of clinical signs, to

Table 1
Commonly used injectable antibiotic combinations for synovial sepsis

	Route	Dose	Frequency
Potassium Penicillin, or	IV—slowly	22,000 IU/kg	Every 6 h
Procaine Penicillin, with	IM	22,000 IU/kg	Every 12 h
Gentamicin	IV	6.6 mg/kg	Every 24 h
Potassium Penicillin, or	IV—slowly	22,000 IU/kg	Every 6 h
Procaine Penicillin, with	IM	22,000 IU/kg	Every 12 h
Amikacin	IV	15–25 mg/kg	Every 24 h
Cefazolin, and	IV	11 mg/kg	Every 8 h
Gentamicin, or	IV	6.6 mg/kg	Every 24 h
Ceftiofur	IV or IM	1 mg/lb	Every 12 h
Enrofloxacin	IV	5–7.5 mg/kg	Every 24 h

Abbreviations: IM, intramuscular; IV, intravenous.

Table 2			
Commonly used oral antibiotic combinations for synovial sepsis			
	Route	Dose	Frequency
Trimethoprim/sulfa (960 mg)	Oral	15 mg/lb	Every 12 h
Doxycycline	Oral	11 mg/kg	Every 12 h
Minocycline	Oral	4 mg/kg	Every 12 h
Enrofloxacin	Oral	7.5 mg/kg	Every 24 h

ensure infection is completely eliminated and recurrence of sepsis is minimized.[5,8] In addition, if there is no growth on bacterial culture or if the sensitivity and specificity are inconclusive, broad-spectrum antibiotics are recommended for 2 to 4 weeks following clinical sign resolution and normalization of synovial fluid parameters.[5]

Local and regional antibiotic administration techniques include intrasynovial injection, regional limb perfusion, continuous rate infusion into the synovial structure, or antibiotic-impregnated delivery systems.[2,11] Intrasynovial antibiotic administration results in elevated concentrations of antibiotic drugs and is performed via synoviocentesis, which must be repeated during the course of treatment.[2] Broad spectrum, concentration-dependent antibiotics are primarily used for the treatment of synovial and orthopedic infections, and aminoglycosides are frequently administered.[7,35,36] However, the results of synovial fluid bacterial culture and sensitivity testing can help determine the most appropriate, case-dependent antibiotic selection.[36]

An alternative to repeated synoviocentesis is the use of specialized infusion systems. These systems are attached to a catheter placed within the affected synovial structure and can facilitate repeated administration or the continuous infusion of an antibiotic.[5,37] Continuous antibiotic infusion can be administered via an intrasynovial catheter attached to a "balloon" continuous rate infusion system, and the continuous rate antibiotic infusion helps maintain the minimal inhibitory concentration (MIC) of the antibiotic in the synovial fluid for longer durations than systemic antibiotic administration alone.[5,38] These systems require asepsis and extensive management to prevent intrasynovial catheter kinking, leakage, or other catheter site complications. These techniques may be beneficial for cases that require repeated intrasynovial treatments.[37]

Regional perfusion of antibiotics can be performed via intravenous or intraosseous routes. Regional antibiotic administration can result in synovial fluid antibiotic concentrations that exceed MIC during the 24 hours after drug administration.[8,39] Regional intravenous perfusions are frequently used for treatment of distal limb wounds in horses. These perfusions are performed via a peripheral vein within a selected portion of the limb distal to a preplaced tourniquet (**Fig. 4**).[36]

The selected antibiotic should be diluted in a solution to create the perfusate, with final perfusate volumes ranging from 10 to 60 mL.[36,40] Although the ideal perfusate volume is unknown, the volume of tissue to be perfused helps determine the final perfusate volume, and volumes of 30 to 60 mL are commonly used for equine distal limb regional perfusions.[4,36,40] After tourniquet application, antibiotic solution is slowly infused into the vein, and the tourniquet is maintained for 20 to 30 minutes to allow the medication to remain within the isolated area.[3,8] As movement of the horse can result in failure of vascular occlusion by the tourniquet and leakage of the perfused antibiotic into the systemic circulation, sedation and appropriate patient restraint is advised.[41] Wide tourniquets, such as Esmarch bandages (Medline, Northfield, IL) or pneumatic tourniquets, provide appropriate vascular occlusion, helping to maintain

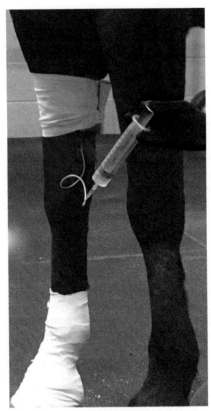

Fig. 4. An Esmarch tourniquet placed above the carpus isolates the distal limb during a regional limb perfusion. The butterfly catheter is inserted in the cephalic vein.

the antibiotic's concentration higher than the MIC within the synovial fluid.[42] Regional perfusion is usually repeated every 24 to 48 hours, and 3 sequential treatments are typically recommended, but additional treatments may be necessary.[8]

Intraosseous regional limb perfusions are performed by drilling a unicortical hole in the bone immediately proximal or distal to the affected joint.[5,43] An intraosseous bone port or temporary tubing is inserted into the hole, allowing antibiotic solutions to be administered directly into the medullary cavity of the bone.[5,43] A tourniquet is placed proximal to the site of administration to help concentrate the antibiotic during perfusion. Intravenous regional limb perfusion is easier to perform and requires less specialized equipment than intraosseous perfusion; however, the intraosseous technique can be used when soft tissue trauma, cellulitis, or vascular damage precludes intravenous perfusion.[8] Intravenous and intraosseous regional limb perfusions result in similar synovial fluid antibiotic concentrations.[43]

Bioabsorbable, or nonabsorbable, antibiotic-impregnated delivery systems (implants) are another way to reach high levels of antibiotic concentration at the site of application.[8,44] One nonabsorbable implant material is polymethylmethacrylate (PMMA), which is a high-density polymer to which antimicrobial drugs can be added, and the mixture is formed into beads or cylinders.[8,45] The local concentration of antibiotic released from PMMA can be up to 200 times greater than that achieved by systemic antibiotic administration. Approximately 5% of the antibiotic solution is released from PMMA within the first 24 to 48 hours after implantation. This is followed by a slow release of the remaining antibiotic over years.[45] PMMA implants can be placed in periarticular tissue and are often removed after 2 to 4 weeks.[5,8] If left in place, PMMA implants can result in localized inflammation or bacterial resistance. PMMA implants should not be placed within a synovial structure, because they induce synovitis and superficial cartilage damage.[5,8,44–46]

Bioabsorbable materials have advantages over PMMA implants because they have a faster and more constant release of antibiotics, better biocompatibility, and biodegradability.[5,47] Chitosan, microspheres, plaster of paris, hydroxyapatite, and collagen-based systems are successfully used bioabsorbable materials.[5,8,44] Gentamicin-impregnated collaged sponges placed intraarticularly after arthroscopic lavage in horses with septic arthritis have resulted in excellent clinical outcomes and may stimulate wound healing.[44,48]

Synovial Lavage and Debridement

The physical removal of inflammatory mediators, devitalized tissue, debris, bacteria, and fibrin from infected synovial structures is one of the most important treatment goals for horses with septic synovitis.[4,5] These materials disturb synovial function and metabolism, which can lead to irreversible joint damage, osteoarthritis, tenosynovitis, and bursitis.[4,11] Synovial lavage and drainage can be performed with through-and-through lavage with hypodermic needles, arthroscopy/tenoscopy, and open incision.[5,7,8,11] Through-and-through lavage is inexpensive and easy to perform under general anesthesia or with standing sedation.[12] Three to five liters of isotonic fluids are recommended and administered through large (usually 18–14 gauge) ingress and egress needles that have been aseptically placed into the affected synovial structure (**Fig. 5**).[11,12,49] If needles become obstructed with fibrin or debris, a stab arthrotomy may be necessary for fluid egress.[11,12] The wound itself can also serve as an egress portal. Through-and-through lavage is frequently used for acute synovial infection, before the development of substantial fibrin deposition. This technique does not allow for the removal of large fibrin clots, foreign material, assessment of the articular cartilage, or the debridement of bone or soft tissue lesions.[3,49]

Arthroscopic lavage is often the preferred treatment, because it allows for directed removal of fibrin or foreign material, visualization of synovial structures, and debridement of bone or soft tissue lesions (**Fig. 6**).[4,5,10,49] Visualization of an affected synovial structure and articular cartilage helps determine the prognosis. Osteomyelitis, osteochondral lesions, and marked deposits of pannus are associated with nonsurvival.[10,49] Overall, arthroscopic evaluation and treatment can decrease the duration of systemic antibiotic administration and decrease the length of hospitalization.[5,10]

Arthrotomy into the distal aspect of a joint can provide surgical access and drainage.[8,49] When combined with systemic and local antibiotics and joint lavage, arthrotomy can successfully resolve infection in cases that have been unresponsive to other treatment methods.[34] Arthrotomy incisions must be appropriately managed to prevent further contamination of the joint. Incisions can be surgically closed or left open to heal by second intention depending on case progression.[34] Although rare, complications associated with arthrotomy include secondary joint infection, joint capsule fibrosis, delayed incision healing, and decreased range of motion.[34] Similar complications can occur in tendon sheaths and bursae. Arthroscopic lavage combined with systemic and local antimicrobial administration is a very effective treatment method, so the need for arthrotomy is not common.[3,49]

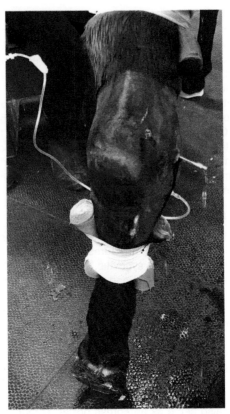

Fig. 5. Through-and-through lavage of the tibiotarsal joint. An 18-gauge needle was aseptically placed into the dorsal aspect of the tibiotarsal joint and pressurized sterile, isotonic fluids were lavaged through the joint. Fluid can be visualized exiting a teat cannula placed within the wound.

Additional Therapies

Septic synovitis typically creates substantial pain. Surgical and antimicrobial treatments help improve comfort in affected horses.[5,11] Maintaining comfort and weight bearing can lead to improved ambulation and joint motion, decreased formation of fibrous adhesions, improved articular cartilage nutrition, and a reduced risk for supporting limb laminitis.[7,49] Nonsteroidal antiinflammatory medications provide analgesia and reduce inflammation, with phenylbutazone, flunixin meglumine, or firocoxib being commonly used.[5,7,50] Alternative methods of analgesia include constant rate intravenous infusions of lidocaine, opioids, or ketamine, epidural analgesia for severe hind limb pain, or topically applied antiinflammatory medications such as diclofenac[5] (see R. Reid Hanson's article, "Medical Therapy in Equine Wound Management," in this issue).

Local and systemic medications directed at enhancing synovial fluid character may be useful additional treatments. However, the status of a septic process and timing of administration are important to determine. Intraarticular polysulfated glycosaminoglycan (PSGAG) and corticosteroids can increase the risk of synovial infection and should not be used during active sepsis.[7,49,51] Intraarticular PSGAG can bind local

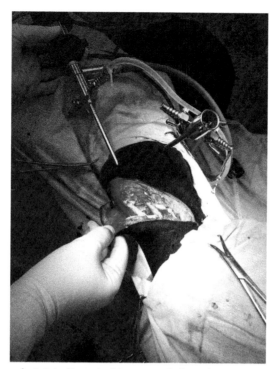

Fig. 6. Arthroscopy of a joint affected with a wound allows for visualization of the synovial structures, lavage, and debridement of associated lesions.

complement, which can reduce the inoculum required to establish sepsis and retard resolution of compartmental infection.[52] Intraarticular hyaluronan can be used for its antiinflammatory effects on septic synovial structures; however, the synovial inflammation may degrade the hyaluronan before it exerting desired effects.[49] To reduce the risk of secondary inflammation or infection, intrasynovial administration of these agents should be performed no sooner than 2 weeks after the resolution of a synovial infection.[49] The systemic administration of hyaluronan (intravenously) or PSGAG (intramuscularly) may provide the most benefit with reduced risk for septic synovial structures.[7,49]

Prognosis

Up to 85% of horses affected with septic synovial structures survive and 33% to 77% of these horses return to athletic function.[1,9,10,49,53] One report found that horses with open wounds involving a synovial structure that were treated medically or surgically within 24 hours of injury were less likely to develop septic arthritis, more likely to survive, and more likely to return to function than horses that were treated more than 24 hours after joint injury occurred.[9] In this clinical report, 53% of horses with open wounds in joints that were treated within 24 hours of injury developed septic arthritis, and these horses had a 65% survival rate.[9] Ninety-two percent of the horses that were treated 2 to 7 days following open joint injury developed septic arthritis, with only 39% of these horses surviving.[9] Therefore, timely diagnosis and treatment of wounds involving synovial structures is critical for obtaining a successful outcome in affected horses.[2]

REFERENCES

1. Schneider R, Bramlage L, Moore R, et al. A retrospective study of 192 horses affected with septic arthritis/tenosynovitis. Equine Vet J 1992;24:436–42.
2. Ludwig EK. Equine septic arthritis and serum amyloid A. Virginia Tech; 2016.
3. Baxter GM. Management of wounds involving synovial structures in horses. Clin Tech Equine Pract 2004;3:204–14.
4. Joyce J. Injury to synovial structures. Vet Clin North Am Equine Pract 2007;23: 103–16.
5. Morton AJ. Diagnosis and treatment of septic arthritis. Vet Clin North Am Equine Pract 2005;21:627–49.
6. Lugo J, Gaughan EM. Septic arthritis, tenosynovitis, and infections of hoof structures. Vet Clin North Am Equine Pract 2006;22:363–88.
7. Bertone AL. Infectious arthritis. In: McIlwraith CW, Trotter GW, editors. Joint disease in the horse. 1st edition. Philadelphia: WB Saunders; 1996. p. 397–409.
8. Carstanjen B, Boehart S, Cislakova M. Septic arthritis in adult horses. Pol J Vet Sci 2010;13:201.
9. Gibson K, McIlwraith C, Turner A, et al. Open joint injuries in horses: 58 cases (1980-1986). J Am Vet Med Assoc 1989;194:398–404.
10. Wright I, Smith M, Humphrey D, et al. Endoscopic surgery in the treatment of contaminated and infected synovial cavities. Equine Vet J 2003;35:613–9.
11. van Weeren PR. Septic arthritis. In: McIlwraith CW, Frisbie DD, Kawcak CE, et al, editors. Joint disease in the horse. 2nd edition. St Louis (MO): Elsevier; 2016. p. 91–104.
12. Richardson DW, Ahern BJ. Synovial and osseous infection. In: Auer JA, Stick JA, editors. Equine surgery. 4th edition. St Louis (MO): Elsevier; 2012. p. 1189–200.
13. van Weeren PR. General anatomy and physiology of joints. In: McIlwraith CW, Frisbie DD, Kawcak CE, et al, editors. Joint disease in the horse. 2nd edition. St Louis (MO): Elsevier; 2016. p. 1–24.
14. McIlwraith CW. General pathobiology of the joint and response to injury. In: McIlwraith CW, Trotter GW, editors. Joint disease in the horse. 1st edition. Philadelphia: WB Saunders; 1996. p. 40–70.
15. Frisbie DD. Synovial joint biology and pathobiology. In: Auer JA, Stick JA, editors. Equine surgery. 4th edition. St. Louis (MO): Elsevier; 2012. p. 1096–113.
16. American Association of Equine Practitioners A. Guide for veterinary service and judging of equestrian events. 4th edition. Lexington (KY): AAEP; 1991.
17. Ludwig EK, Wiese RB, Graham MR, et al. Serum and synovial fluid serum amyloid A response in equine models of synovitis and septic arthritis. Vet Surg 2016;45: 859–67.
18. Beccati F, Gialletti R, Passamonti F, et al. Ultrasonographic findings in 38 horses with septic arthritis/tenosynovitis. Vet Radiol Ultrasound 2015;56:68–76.
19. Easley JT, Brokken MT, Zubrod CJ, et al. Magnetic resonance imaging findings in horses with septic arthritis. Vet Radiol Ultrasound 2011;52:402–8.
20. Steel CM. Equine synovial fluid analysis. Vet Clin North Am Equine Pract 2008;24: 437–54.
21. Todhunter RJ. General principles of joint pathobiology. In: McIlwraith CW, Trotter GW, editors. Joint disease in the horse. 1st edition. Philadelphia: WB Saunders; 1996. p. 1–28.
22. Bertone AL. Update on infectious arthritis in horses. Equine Vet Educ 1999;11: 143–52.

23. Van Pelt R. Interpretation of synovial fluid findings in the horse. J Am Vet Med Assoc 1974;165:91–5.

24. Madison J, Sommer M, Spencer P. Relations among synovial membrane histopathologic findings, synovial fluid cytologic findings, and bacterial culture results in horses with suspected infectious arthritis: 64 cases (1979-1987). J Am Vet Med Assoc 1991;198:1655–61.

25. Taylor AH, Mair TS, Smith LJ, et al. Bacterial culture of septic synovial structures of horses: does a positive bacterial culture influence prognosis? Equine Vet J 2010;42:213–8.

26. Montgomery R, Long I, Milton J, et al. Comparison of aerobic culturette, synovial membrane biopsy, and blood culture medium in detection of canine bacterial arthritis. Vet Surg 1989;18:300–3.

27. Dechant JE, Symm WA, Nieto JE. Comparison of pH, lactate, and glucose analysis of equine synovial fluid using a portable clinical analyzer with a bench-top blood gas analyzer. Vet Surg 2011;40:811–6.

28. Tulamo R, Bramlage L, Gabel A. Sequential clinical and synovial fluid changes associated with acute infectious arthritis in the horse. Equine Vet J 1989;21:325–31.

29. Jacobsen S, Thomsen MH, Nanni S. Concentrations of serum amyloid A in serum and synovial fluid from healthy horses and horses with joint disease. Am J Vet Res 2006;67:1738–42.

30. Pepys M, Baltz ML, Tennent GA, et al. Serum amyloid A protein (SAA) in horses: objective measurement of the acute phase response. Equine Vet J 1989;21:106–9.

31. Jacobsen S, Andersen P. The acute phase protein serum amyloid A (SAA) as a marker of inflammation in horses. Equine Vet Educ 2007;19:38–46.

32. Uhlar CM, Whitehead AS. Serum amyloid A, the major vertebrate acute-phase reactant. Eur J Biochem 1999;265:501–23.

33. McDonald TL, Larson MA, Mack DR, et al. Elevated extrahepatic expression and secretion of mammary-associated serum amyloid A 3 (M-SAA3) into colostrum. Vet Immunol Immunopathol 2001;83:203–11.

34. Schneider R, Bramlage L, Mecklenburg LM, et al. Open drainage, intra-articular and systemic antibiotics in the treatment of septic arthritis/tenosynovitis in horses. Equine Vet J 1992;24:443–9.

35. Zantingh AJ, Schwark WS, Fubini SL, et al. Accumulation of amikacin in synovial fluid after regional limb perfusion of amikacin sulfate alone and in combination with ticarcillin/clavulanate in horses. Vet Surg 2014;43:282–8.

36. Rubio-Martínez LM, Cruz AM. Antimicrobial regional limb perfusion in horses. J Am Vet Med Assoc 2006;228:706–12, 655.

37. Stewart A, Goodrich L, Byron C, et al. Antimicrobial delivery by intrasynovial catheterisation with systemic administration for equine synovial trauma and sepsis. Aust Vet J 2010;88:115–23.

38. Lescun TB, Vasey JR, Ward MP, et al. Treatment with continuous intrasynovial antimicrobial infusion for septic synovitis in horses: 31 cases (2000–2003). J Am Vet Med Assoc 2006;228:1922–9.

39. Werner LA, Hardy J, Bertone AL. Bone gentamicin concentration after intra-articular injection or regional intravenous perfusion in the horse. Vet Surg 2003;32:559–65.

40. Hyde RM, Lynch TM, Clark CK, et al. The influence of perfusate volume on antimicrobial concentration in synovial fluid following intravenous regional limb perfusion in the standing horse. Can Vet J 2013;54:363.

41. Mahne AT, Rioja E, Marais HJ, et al. Clinical and pharmacokinetic effects of regional or general anaesthesia on intravenous regional limb perfusion with amikacin in horses. Equine Vet J 2014;46:375–9.
42. Levine DG, Epstein KL, Ahern BJ, et al. Efficacy of three tourniquet types for intravenous antimicrobial regional limb perfusion in standing horses. Vet Surg 2010; 39:1021–4.
43. Butt TD, Bailey JV, Dowling PM, et al. Comparison of 2 techniques for regional antibiotic delivery to the equine forelimb: intraosseous perfusion vs. intravenous perfusion. Can Vet J 2001;42:617.
44. Haerdi-Landerer MC, Habermacher J, Wenger B, et al. Slow release antibiotics for treatment of septic arthritis in large animals. Vet J 2010;184:14–20.
45. Sayegh AI, Moore RM. Polymethylmethacrylate beads for treating orthopedic infections. Compendium on Continuing Education for the Practicing Veterinarian 2003;25:788–95.
46. Farnsworth KD, White NA, Robertson J. The effect of implanting gentamicin-impregnated polymethylmethacrylate beads in the tarsocrural joint of the horse. Vet Surg 2001;30:126–31.
47. Miclau T, Dahners LE, Lindsey RW. In vitro pharmacokinetics of antibiotic release from locally implantable materials. J Orthop Res 1993;11:627–32.
48. Summerhays G. Treatment of traumatically induced synovial sepsis in horses with gentamicin-impregnated collagen sponges. Vet Rec 2000;147:184–8.
49. Baxter GM. Diagnosis and management of wounds involving synovial structures. In: Stashak TS, Theoret C, editors. Equine wound management. 2nd edition. Ames (IA): Blackwell; 2008. p. 463–88.
50. Palmer JL, Bertone AL. Joint structure, biochemistry and biochemical disequilibrium in synovitis and equine joint disease. Equine Vet J 1994;26:263–77.
51. Gustafson S, McIlwraith C, Jones R. Comparison of the effect of polysulfated glycosaminoglycan, corticosteroids, and sodium hyaluronate in the potentiation of a subinfective dose of Staphylococcus aureus in the midcarpal joint of horses. Am J Vet Res 1989;50:2014–7.
52. Rashmir-Raven AM, Coyne CP, Fenwick BW, et al. Inhibition of equine complement activity by polysulfated glycosaminoglycans. Am J Vet Res 1992;53:87–90.
53. Walmsley E, Anderson G, Muurlink M, et al. Retrospective investigation of prognostic indicators for adult horses with infection of a synovial structure. Aust Vet J 2011;89:226–31.

Medical Therapy in Equine Wound Management

R. Reid Hanson, DVM

KEYWORDS

- Equine • Wounds • Antibiotics • Regional limb perfusion • Intraosseous perfusion
- Antibiotic-impregnated polymethylmethacrylate beads

KEY POINTS

- Acute superficial wound infections are usually the result of one dominating microorganism, whereas chronic or deep wound infections of horses are often polymicrobial.
- The most common organisms for subcutaneous tissue wounds are *Staphylococcus* species, which tend to be deceptive in onset and provoke a chronic inflammatory response.
- Traumatic synovial structure wound infections are typically gram-negative enteric genera, *Streptococcus*, and *Staphylococcus*. Polymicrobial infection is common.
- Regional and intraosseous perfusion maximizes efficacy of antibiotics by concentrating the antibiotic in a confined area to promote a concentration gradient.
- Antibiotic-impregnated polymethylmethacrylate beads are predominantly helpful for wounds that have a poor blood supply and for wounds containing surgical implants that must remain in place.

INTRODUCTION

The primary objective for the medical management of wounds is preventing infection and creating an optimum environment for wound healing with the reestablishment of an epithelial cover and recovery of tissue integrity, strength, and function. The goal in antimicrobial therapy is to administer an appropriate drug regimen so that pathogens are killed or curbed to the extent that they are purged by the host's immune system and no longer impede wound healing. The appropriate drug is determined by identifying the principal pathogens within the wound and associated antibiotic sensitivities. Regrettably, inappropriate use of antibiotics is likely a major cause for the widespread emergence of resistant pathogenic bacterial organisms.[1,2]

Disclosure Statement: The author has no financial or personal relationship with other people or organizations that could inappropriately influence or bias the content of the article.
Department of Clinical Sciences, J.T. Vaughan Teaching Hospital, Auburn University College of Veterinary Medicine, Auburn, AL 36849, USA
E-mail address: hansorr@auburn.edu

Vet Clin Equine 34 (2018) 591–603
https://doi.org/10.1016/j.cveq.2018.07.008
0749-0739/18/© 2018 Elsevier Inc. All rights reserved.

PROPHYLACTIC USE OF ANTIBIOTICS

Administration of prophylactic antibiotics to horses undergoing a clean surgical procedure of short duration is not indicated, except when the development of a surgical site infection (SSI) would be performance limiting or life threatening.[3] Although many factors contribute to SSI, studies suggest that the incidence of infection in horses after clean surgical procedures is very low.[4,5] Horses that have elective arthroscopy without receiving perioperative prophylactic antibiotics have a 0.5% incidence of septic arthritis versus a 0.9% incidence for horses undergoing arthroscopy that receive antibiotics perioperatively.[4,5] However, antimicrobial prophylaxis is indicated if the equine surgical patient is at high risk of infection; that is, when the likelihood of occurrence of infection exceeds 5% without prophylactic antimicrobial use.[3]

The use of antimicrobial drugs should not replace meticulous aseptic and atraumatic surgical technique. These include atraumatic handling of tissue, good hemostasis, preservation of blood supply, strict aseptic technique, accurate apposition and minimum tension on tissue, use of appropriately sized suture material, and obliteration of dead space. Risk factors of infection include surgical procedures that are clean-contaminated or contaminated, surgical times that exceed 60 minutes, anesthetic plane depths that may affect perfusion and oxygenation of tissues, and the presence of orthopedic implants.[6–12]

Suitable use of prophylactic antimicrobial drugs depends on the accurate selection of appropriate antibiotics, dosing regimen, and duration of use. An antibiotic with a narrow spectrum of activity should be selected for use to preserve the patient's normal flora and decrease the risk for development of antimicrobial resistance. Prophylactic antimicrobial therapy should begin preoperatively so that the concentrations of the drug in serum and tissues lasts for the duration of surgery and exceeds the minimum inhibitory concentration for organisms likely to be encountered.[13,14] The current recommendation is for the preoperative dose to be administered within 60 minutes of skin incision and for readministering during surgery if the procedure extends beyond 2 half-lives of the antibiotic.[14] The antibiotics used prophylactically most commonly in equine medicine, penicillin and gentamicin, reach peak concentrations at the surgical site between 15 and 30 minutes after intravenous (IV) administration, with concentrations declining rapidly thereafter.[15–17] The half-life of potassium penicillin G (20,000 IU/kg, IV) in horses is approximately 40 minutes, whereas that of gentamicin sulfate (6.6 mg/kg, IV) is approximately 90 minutes.[15–17]

For humans, prophylactic antibiotic therapy should be continued for no more than 24 hours postoperatively irrespective of whether the surgery was clean, clean-contaminated, or contaminated.[18–20] Prolonged administration of prophylactic antibiotics can result in increased morbidity, including a 33% greater rate of hospital infection, a 15% greater incidence of surgical wound infection, and may contribute to antimicrobial resistance.[18–20] There is no difference in the rate of SSI between horses that received antibiotics for less than 36 hours after exploratory celiotomy versus horses treated more than 36 hours, nor is there a benefit in administrating antibiotics for 120 hours rather than 72 hours, to prevent incisional infections after surgery for an acute abdominal crisis.[21,22]

THERAPEUTIC USE OF ANTIBIOTICS

Systemic administration of antibiotics is warranted when the degree of infection exceeds the efforts of local control of the bioburden and signs of local soft tissue infection or systemic infection are apparent.[23] Because the indication for systemic antibiotic therapy is not always clear, antimicrobial drugs are often administered empirically, as a routine adjunct to the management of open wounds or when the wound is at high risk of becoming infected, such as with puncture wounds, devitalized tissue, open fractures, or has entered a body cavity or a synovial structure[24–26] (see Elsa K. Ludwig and Philip D. van Harreveld's article, "Wounds Over Synovial Structures," and Randy B. Eggleston's article, "Wound Management: Wounds With Special Challenges," in this issue).

A long delay between the onset of injury and treatment increases the risk that contamination will progress to colonization and infection. Debridement, irrigation, and topical therapies are fundamental to reducing the bacterial burden and disrupting biofilms (see Karl E. Frees' article, "Equine Practice on Wound Management: Wound Cleansing and Hygiene," and Britta S. Leise's article, "Topical Wound Medications," in this issue). Bacteria that become embedded in an extracellular polymeric substance (biofilm) are slow or nongrowing, but can delay wound healing because bacteria in biofilms have enhanced virulence, are protected from the immune response of the host, and are more likely resistant to antimicrobials.[27]

Bacteria cultured from acute and chronic wounds show a significantly higher potential for biofilm formation than bacteria isolated from skin. *Pseudomonas aeruginosa* and *Enterococcus faecium* are the bacteria species most commonly isolated from equine wound and skin samples, respectively. *Staphylococcus* was the most commonly isolated genus isolated from either environment.[28] Although bacterial colonization of a wound does not necessarily prevent wound healing, the presence of multiple bacterial species capable of biofilm formation suggests that bacteria may be surviving and proliferating within biofilm and subsequently hindering wound healing.[28,29]

Ideally, a wound exudate for bacterial culture and antibiotic sensitivity testing should be collected before instituting therapy. The sample should be harvested from deep within the wound rather than from its contaminated surface.[30] This enables targeting the microorganisms with a narrow-spectrum antimicrobial drug. Selected antibiotics should reflect the microbial predilection while considering the prevalence of antimicrobial resistance and the importance of using a narrow-spectrum antibiotic based on antibiotic sensitivity testing of bacterial isolates.[28,31,32] If clinical signs of infection evolve, final selection of the antibiotic is based on the results of culture and sensitivity tests.

For wounds of subcutaneous tissue, the most commonly cultured organisms are *Staphyloccus* sp, which tend to be insidious in colonization and provoke a chronic inflammatory response.[33,34] The less commonly found organisms involved in wound infection are *Streptococcus,* gram-negative aerobes, anaerobes, and *Corynebacterium pseudotuberculosis*. Penicillin, or trimethoprim-sulfonamide, or a combination of both, are often used empirically to treat acute or superficial wound infections while awaiting results of culture and sensitivity. Puncture wounds, including those involving synovial cavities, are frequently best treated with a beta-lactam antibiotic along with an aminoglycoside, such as gentamicin sulfate or amikacin sulfate because infections are often polymicrobial.[22–26,28,30–33] Ceftiofur sodium or enrofloxacin are generally reserved for infections resistant to penicillin and aminoglycosides.[22,33] Enrofloxacin is not recommended for use in young horses because it can rapidly lead to noninflammatory arthropathy in immature animals.[35] High doses of penicillin and metronidazole are recommended for treating deep fascial cellulitis, septic myositis, or pyonecrotic processes associated with *Clostridium* sp.[22,32] Antibiotic treatment of clostridial infection is typically required for weeks and discontinuation is based on the health of the affected tissues and negative culture results. *S* sp infections typically are more antibiotic sensitive, so treatment is commonly shorter (10–14 days).

Wounds of muscle typically respond very well to antimicrobial therapy, needing only a short course of treatment. Open drainage of muscle wounds, which is not difficult at most sites, speeds resolution of infection particularly with intramuscular abscesses. Clostridial myonecrosis can rapidly cause severe systemic illness but with aggressive surgical debridement and aeration, local and systemic antibiotic therapy often resolves infection within days.[33]

For traumatic wounds of a synovial structure complicated by infection, the most commonly cultured organisms are gram-negative enteric genera, *Streptococcus* and *Staphylococcus*. Polymicrobial infection is common[33,35] (see Elsa K. Ludwig and Philip D. van Harreveld's article, "Wounds Over Synovial Structures," in this issue). Postoperative infection of a synovial structure typically involves *Staphylococcus, Streptococcus, Enterobacter, Pseudomonas*, or other enteric genera.[33,35] Administration of both a cephalosporin and gentamicin or amikacin is indicated for treatment of an infected synovial structure; enrofloxacin alone is a reasonable alternative in adult horses.[32] Metronidazole may be additionally administered for wounds on the distal aspect of the limb or other wounds likely to have fecal contamination or the presence of obligate anaerobes. Synovial structures usually require treatment for weeks using parenterally administered antibiotics initially that may be switched to oral administration after substantial improvement is seen. Intrasynovial lavage and antibiotic infusion are indicated and repeated, if needed. Regional perfusion for wounds at or distal to the carpus or tarsus is indicated and repeated, if needed.[36]

Traumatic wounds involving bone or physeal cartilage typically involve *Enterobacter, Streptococcus, Staphylococcus,* and in young foals, gram-negative enteric genera[33] (see Randy B. Eggleston's article, "Wound Management: Wounds With Special Challenges," in this issue). For postoperative osseous infections, *Streptococcus zooepidemicus, Staphylococcus aureus,* or another *Streptococcus* species is most commonly isolated.[9] The antibiotic treatment options are the same as for synovial structures. Weeks or months of antibiotic therapy is usually required for resolution of infection of bone or physeal cartilage.

The intravenous route should be used initially for systemic administration of antibiotics because the desired serum concentration of a drug is more predictable than when the drug is administered by other routes. The antibiotic can be administered orally or intramuscularly after an adequate concentration of the drug in the blood has been achieved by intravenous administration. Regional intravenous perfusion is particularly useful in the management of infected wounds on the distal aspect of limbs of horses, as it provides a high concentration of the antimicrobial drug at the target. Multiple surgical debridements of a wound may be necessary. The implantation of antibiotic-impregnated polymethylmethacrylate (PMMA) beads into a wound are particularly important when complete debridement is not possible or when surgical implants must remain.[36]

The duration of treatment of any wound infection is primarily dictated by the patient's response to therapy. The benchmarks that indicate a positive response include resolution of systemic signs of inflammation, continued improvement in comfort and function, reduction and ultimately resolution of the localized signs of inflammation and purulent discharge, negative culture result, and a normal rate of wound healing. Administration of antimicrobial drugs should not be continued once there is clinical and microbiologic evidence that an infection has been eliminated.[37]

REGIONAL INTRAVENOUS ANTIBIOTIC DELIVERY

Regional intravenous delivery of antibiotics may be pivotal for resolution of well-established infections, wounds of inadequately perfused tissue, biofilm-infected wounds, and wounds involving surgical implants that must remain in place. Targeted modes of antibiotic delivery may even preclude the need for systemic antibiotic therapy in certain cases.

Regional intravenous limb perfusion with antibiotics maximizes efficacy of treatment while minimizing the cost of the drug and the risks of toxicity and development of antibiotic resistance. Therapeutic concentrations of antibiotic can be achieved even in poorly perfused wounds or those with necrotic tissue, because the drug diffuses down a concentration gradient from the vascular space to the interstitial space. Regional intravenous perfusion is most effective with concentration-dependent antibiotics, such as aminoglycosides, although it may also be effective with time-dependent antibiotics, such as penicillins and cephalosporins. For susceptible pathogens, a single treatment may be adequate when administered in concert with systemic antimicrobial therapy.[38]

As most regional intravenous limb perfusions are usually performed in the standing horse, the patient should be sedated and the site of catheter placement desensitized with regional anesthesia. A palmar nerve block for digital perfusion via a palmar digital vein improves patient comfort and reduces movement during perfusion. A ring block may be used for regions with complicated or multifaceted innervation. The level of sedation necessary is dictated by the horse's temperament and severity of pain and achieved by choice and dose of the sedative.

To prepare for regional intravenous limb perfusion, the skin should be clipped and aseptically prepared, as for a routine IV catheterization. A sterile IV catheter, such as a butterfly, or short over-the-needle catheter, is used for a single treatment. It is convenient to use an indwelling IV catheter for repeated treatment. Catheter gauge and length vary according to vein diameter and shape. An extension set can be affixed to the hub of the catheter, which is glued or taped to the skin with adhesive tape. It is best to place and secure the catheter before applying the tourniquet, because securing the catheter may take several minutes and the tourniquet must be removed 30 minutes after placement.

Tourniquets limit the antibiotic to the perfused area, thereby creating local concentrations of the antibiotic in tissues and fluids that significantly exceed those achieved after systemic administration. An Esmarch or pneumatic tourniquet is applied firmly and then secured so that it occludes venous outflow for the duration of the 30-minute procedure.[39,40] Adhesive tape or a bandage should be applied to secure the Esmarch bandage after application.

Where possible, a pair of tourniquets proximal and distal to the wound and catheter/cannula site should be used to isolate the infected area and nearby vein. Narrow rubber tourniquets and elastic bandages are not suitable for this procedure.[39] The proximal tourniquet prevents escape of the antibiotic into the systemic circulation during perfusion. The distal tourniquet limits the volume of tissue being perfused. A tourniquet that is applied too lightly or that loosens allows the antibiotic to exit the area and escape into systemic circulation before the procedure is completed, which prevents achieving locally high antibiotic concentrations at the site of the infection. If using a palmar/plantar digital vein for IV perfusion, the tourniquet should be applied in the mid-metacarpal/tarsal region. If using the cephalic/saphenous vein because of local swelling distally, apply the tourniquet to the distal aspect of the radius/tibia.

The antibiotic solution should be immediately infused after applying the tourniquets. To reduce the hydrostatic pressure during infusion, and reduce the risk of extravascular leakage and perivascular inflammation, blood is allowed to flow without restrictions from the extension set until it slows to a drip, or alternatively, a volume of blood equal to the intended infusion can be aspirated. The antibiotic solution is infused slowly over 1 to 2 minutes, then the drug within the extension set is emptied into the catheter by infusing a small bolus of air.

The tourniquet is removed after 30 minutes. The catheter is removed unless repeated perfusion is anticipated. Firm digital pressure is applied to the venipuncture site or the site is securely wrapped for a few minutes. The venipuncture site is then covered with a sterile dressing and light pressure wrap. Maintenance of an indwelling catheter is the same as for IV catheterization at any other site. More perivascular swelling may be present for 24 to 48 hours after catheter removal, but no other adverse effects are seen in most cases. Using a topical nonsteroidal anti-inflammatory drug (NSAID) (eg, 1% diclofenac liposomal cream) may be of value if an indwelling catheter was not placed and the site may need to be used again.[41,42]

The dose of amikacin used is prescribed by the size of the perfused area: 500 to 1000 mg for smaller areas like the digits through the palmar or plantar vein, or 2.0 to 2.5 g when perfusing the distal aspect of the limb via the cephalic or saphenous vein for the carpus or tarsus. Other commonly administered drugs and dosages that can be incorporated into a regional limb perfusion route in an adult horse include gentamicin: 100 to 300 mg; Na/K penicillin: 10 million to 20 million units; ceftiofur: 2 g; enrofloxacin: 700 mg (1.5 mg/kg); and marbofloxacin: 300 mg (0.67 mg/kg). Enrofloxacin may cause vasculitis at therapeutic dosages, so is best reserved for documented enrofloxacin-sensitive infections with no other reasonable options. Bactericidal drugs (eg, aminoglycosides, penicillins, cephalosporins, metronidazole, rifampin, and quinolones in adult horses) are best used to treat severely infected wounds rather than using bacteriostatic drugs (eg, chloramphenicol, tetracyclines, sulfonamides, macrolides, and trimethoprim-sulfonamide combinations).[36,38,42,43]

Volumes commonly administered are 20 to 30 mL for perfusion of the digit via a digital vein; 60 mL for larger areas, such as the carpus/tarsus, distal aspect of the limb; and up to 100 mL for distal limb perfusion via the cephalic/saphenous vein. However, lower perfusion volumes with higher drug concentrations, such as 500 mg gentamicin diluted in 10 mL with sterile isotonic saline solution for perfusion of the distal aspect of the limb via a palmar digital vein may be equally effective.[33,34] Lower perfusion volumes also may reduce the risk of extravascular leakage and perivascular inflammation caused by high hydrostatic pressures associated with larger volumes.[34,44]

A disadvantage of regional limb perfusion with antibiotics is that intravenous perfusion is difficult or impossible when soft tissue swelling obscures the desired vein.[39] There is potential for phlebitis and local tissue necrosis with IV perfusion, particularly when the procedure is repeated or if perivascular leakage occurs. Regional limb perfusion is limited to wounds at or below the carpus or tarsus because a tourniquet must be applied proximal to the site and there is limited residual effect after the tourniquet is removed.[22,39,42]

For intrasynovial injections into a joint space, tendon sheath, or bursa, it is important to use meticulous aseptic technique to avoid further contamination of the synovial structure while injecting an antibiotic. Improved effectiveness of the antibiotic can be achieved if the joint space is lavaged liberally beforehand. Although constant-rate infusion of antibiotic is described for synovial injections in horses, clinical response and long-standing effect seem analogous to individual-dose intrasynovial injection.[45] Commonly administered antibiotics using this route for adult horses include amikacin: 500 to 1000 mg; gentamicin: 150 to 500 mg; ceftiofur: 150 mg; cefazolin: 250 to 500 mg; and Na/K penicillin: 2 million to 5 million units.[38]

INTRAOSSEOUS REGIONAL LIMB PERFUSION

Intraosseous (IO) perfusion is indicated when there is severe soft tissue swelling, edema, or when the veins are not easily accessed. Intraosseous perfusion involves drilling a hole through cortical bone into the medullary cavity. A site is selected that has the greatest and most reachable medullary cavity nearest the wound and that lies just under the skin, requiring little or no surgical dissection to access. The distal aspect of tibia or proximal third of the metatarsus are commonly chosen as sites for IO perfusion of the tarsus. The horse is sedated and the drill site desensitized using regional anesthesia. Hair is clipped and skin is aseptically prepared. Using aseptic technique, a 1-cm incision is made through skin, subcutis, and periosteum over the infusion site, taking care to avoid nerves, vessels, and tendons. The soft tissue is gently retracted with a pair of hemostatic forceps and a 4-mm-diameter uni-cortical hole is drilled through the cortex. The hole is subsequently tapped to 5.5 mm in diameter, if a self-tapping screw is not used, and a 5.5-mm 20-mm cannulated bone screw is inserted so that it provides direct access to the medullary cavity. The male end of a catheter extension set is attached to the Luer lock adapter inserted into the cannulated screw. Alternatively, the male adapter end of an IV delivery set can be carefully wedged into a 4-mm-diameter bone hole.[46]

Tourniquets are applied proximally and distally before antibiotic perfusion to isolate the wound and cannula site to prevent the escape of the infused antibiotic into the systemic circulation. The distal tourniquet limits the volume of tissue being perfused, and thus dilution of the antibiotic in the extracellular fluid. For wounds at or distal to the metacarpo/metatarsophalangeal joint, a single tourniquet is applied proximal to the site. For standing horses, 2 to 3 mL of a local anesthetic solution is infused into the medullary cavity to reduce discomfort caused by the increase in intramedullary pressure during infusion. With tourniquets occluding blood flow proximally and distally, the antibiotic, diluted in 60 mL sterile isotonic saline solution is slowly infused into the medullary cavity over 10 minutes, from where it is absorbed into the regional vasculature. The tourniquet is removed 30 minutes after completing the infusion.

If planning to repeat the IO infusion, the port in the bone screw is capped and covered with a sterile dressing and protective bandage; otherwise the cannulated screw is removed and skin is either closed or left to heal by second intention. In either case, the site is covered with a sterile dressing and light pressure wrap. Localized soft tissue swelling can be expected at the site for a few days after IO perfusion, as can a small amount of serosanguinous discharge when the skin incision is not closed primarily. No treatment other than basic postsurgical wound care is required.

ANTIBIOTIC-IMPREGNATED POLYMETHYLMETHACRYLATE BEADS

Antibiotic-impregnated polymethylmethacrylate (PMMA) beads are predominantly helpful for treatment of wounds that have a poor blood supply and for those containing surgical implants that must remain in place. They may also be useful for treatment of infected wounds in problematic patients that make other forms of antibiotic delivery and wound care challenging or unachievable. Locally high antibiotic concentrations can be sustained in the wound, which may allow discontinuation of systemic antibiotic therapy.[38]

The antibiotic, preferably in lyophilized form, is mixed with the dry PMMA polymer at a rate of 1 to 4 g antibiotic to 20 g polymer. The liquid monomer is applied in a powder-to-liquid ratio of 2:1, and mixed thoroughly for 1 minute. If using a bead mold, 3 strands of size 0 braided polyester suture material can be placed over one-half of the mold, and both halves of the mold are filled with the PMMA mixture. The mold is closed and clamped tightly, allowing the beads to take an appropriate size and spherical or cylindrical shape for the wound and then put aside to harden for at least 10 minutes. A bead mold that forms 6-mm-diameter beads is optimal for treatment of most infected wounds. When using more than one antibiotic, a separate batch of PMMA beads should be made for each drug. Metronidazole may be mixed with hoof acrylic (Equilox; Equilox International, Pine Island, MN) for treatment of polymicrobial infections.[38]

The size and number of antibiotic-impregnated PMMA beads implanted in a wound are determined by the dimensions of a wound. When the beads are placed into the wound, they release sustained therapeutic concentrations of the antibiotic into the surrounding fluid and tissue for several days or weeks. Unless the beads are being implanted while the horse is anesthetized, the horse is sedated and local or regional anesthesia is used to desensitize the wound. The beads may be held in place by partially suturing the wound or by maintaining a sterile dressing over the wound. If the beads are not used immediately after formulation, they should be stored in a sterile, airtight container away from direct light until implanted.

Because the PMMA beads do not biodegrade, they may need to be removed after treatment, depending on the type of wound, ease of the bead removal, and the likelihood of them causing functional impairment if left in place. The beads may be left in place unless they are causing persistent foreign body reaction and drainage, are likely to interfere with future athletic function, or need to be replaced with fresh antibiotic-impregnated beads. Removing the beads can be difficult after approximately 10 days because they become encapsulated by fibrous tissue as the wound heals. Intrasynovial use of PMMA beads is not advised, because it may cause synovial irritation and pain, but if used, the beads should be removed as soon as the infection is resolved, and at most in fewer than 10 days[38] (see Elsa K. Ludwig and Philip D. van Harreveld's article, "Wounds Over Synovial Structures," in this issue).

NONSTEROIDAL ANTI-INFLAMMATORIES

Inflammation is a normal part of the wound-healing process, and is important for the removal of contaminating microorganisms. In the absence of effective decontamination, however, inflammation may be prolonged. Both bacteria and endotoxins can lead to the prolonged elevation of proinflammatory cytokines, such as interleukin (IL)-1 and tumor necrosis factor-α, and lengthen the inflammatory phase leading to chronicity and failure to heal. Prolonged inflammation within a wound also leads to an increased concentration of matrix metalloproteases, a family of proteases that can degrade the extracellular matrix. Accompanied by the increased protease content in a chronically inflamed wound, the concentration of naturally occurring protease inhibitors can decrease. This shift in protease balance in chronic wounds can cause growth factors that promote healing to be rapidly degraded.[47,48]

NSAIDs are commonly administered to wounded horses for the treatment of inflammation and for pain management. These drugs inhibit the activity of cyclooxygenase-1 (COX-1) and cyclooxygenase-2 (COX-2) enzymes and thereby the synthesis of eicosanoids, such as prostaglandins, thromboxanes, and leukotrienes. It is likely that most of the analgesic effects of NSAIDs are related to a reduction in inflammation and swelling without affecting the central nervous system.[49] Selective inhibition of COX-2 enzymes in the horse may provide anti-inflammatory, analgesic, and antipyretic effects without causing adverse effects on the gastrointestinal system, such as right dorsal colitis, which is attributed to COX-1 enzyme inhibition.[49]

Some NSAID drugs are thought to be clinically more effective for ameliorating musculoskeletal pain, and others are believed to be more effective for ameliorating visceral pain. For example, flunixin meglumine is considered to be more effective than phenylbutazone for controlling abdominal, uterine, and ophthalmic pain, whereas phenylbutazone is believed to be more effective in controlling musculoskeletal pain. Nevertheless, flunixin can reduce musculoskeletal inflammation and pain, and phenylbutazone is clinically effective for treatment of visceral pain.[50–53]

There are few data to suggest that short-term administration of NSAID drugs has a negative impact on healing. However, the question of whether long-term administration of NSAID drugs interferes with wound healing remains unanswered. In animal models, systemic use of ibuprofen has demonstrated effects on wound healing that include decreased numbers of fibroblasts, weakened wound breaking strength, reduced wound contraction, delayed epithelialization, and impaired angiogenesis.[54–57] The effects of administering an NSAID drug to equine patients during the early phase of wound healing have not been investigated extensively. One study examining incisional healing found that oxyphenbutazone administered to horses at a loading dose 12 mg/kg for 2 days and then a maintenance dose of 6 mg/kg for 5 days significantly reduced wound inflammation and formation of granulation tissue.[58]

The most common use of NSAIDs is for treatment of musculoskeletal and abdominal pain. The NSAIDs most commonly administered to horses are phenylbutazone, flunixin meglumine, and more recently, the selective COX-2 inhibitors carprofen, meloxicam, and firocoxib.[59] Dosages for NSAIDs commonly used in horses are as follows: phenylbutazone 2.2 to 4.4 mg/kg, every 12 hours, intravenous or oral; flunixin meglumine 0.25 to 1 mg/kg, every 8 to 24 hours, intravenous, oral, or intramuscular; carprofen 0.7 mg/kg, every 24 hours, intravenous or oral; ketoprofen 2.2 mg/kg every 24 hours, intravenous; meloxicam 0.6 mg/kg every 24 hours, oral; or firocoxib 0.1 mg/kg, every 24 hours, oral.[53]

DIMETHYLSULFOXIDE

Dimethylsulfoxide (DMSO) is an effective anti-inflammatory, analgesic, and enzyme activator/inhibitor.[60–62] Significantly decreased white blood cell counts in the synovial fluid of joints with chemically induced synovitis treated with DMSO have been reported.[63] DMSO may also possess some bacteriostatic properties as a result of its effect on the immune response and the reduction of endotoxin-induced tissue damage.[60,62] Increased blood flow through experimental skin flaps and the presence of vascular dilation with DMSO application has also been reported.[62] DMSO appears to assist other treatments in attempts to reduce wound-associated limb edema. A 20% solution using medical-grade 90% DMSO in 250 mL Lactated Ringer's Solution with 1 to 2 g of amikacin added has been described as a perfusate.[64] Such properties provide rationale for its use in conjunction with an antibiotic for regional limb perfusion.

REFERENCES

1. European Wound Management Association. Management of wound infection. London: Medical Education Partnership Ltd.; 2006. p. 1–19.
2. Weese JS, Lefebvre SL. Risk factors for methicillin-resistant *Staphylococcus aureus* colonization in horses admitted to a veterinary teaching hospital. Can Vet J 2007;48:921–6.
3. Southwood LL. Perioperative antimicrobials: should we be concerned about antimicrobial drug use in equine surgical patients. Equine Vet J 2014;46:267–9.

4. Borg H, Carmalt JL. Postoperative septic arthritis after elective equine arthroscopy without antimicrobial prophylaxis. Vet Surg 2013;42:262–6.
5. Olds AM, Stewart AA, Freeman DE, et al. Evaluation of the rate of development of septic arthritis after elective arthroscopy in horses: 7 cases (1994-2003). J Am Vet Med Assoc 2006;229:1949–54.
6. Brown DC, Conzemius MG, Shofer F, et al. Epidemiologic evaluation of postoperative wound infection in dogs and cats. J Am Vet Med Assoc 1997;210:1302–6.
7. Beal MW, Brown DC, Shofer FS. The effects of perioperative hypothermia and the duration of anesthesia on postoperative wound infection rate in clean wounds: a retrospective study. Vet Surg 2000;29:123–7.
8. Wilson DA, Baker GJ, Boero MJ. Complications of celiotomy incisions in horses. Vet Surg 1995;24:506–14.
9. McDonald DG, Morley PS, Bailey JV, et al. An examination of occurrence of surgical wound infection following orthopedic surgery. Equine Vet J 1994;26:323–6.
10. Kotani N, Hashimoto H, Sessler DI, et al. Intraoperative modulation of alveolar macrophages function during isoflurane and propofol anesthesia. Anesthesiology 1998;89:1125–32.
11. Ciepichal J, Kubler A. Effect of general and regional anesthesia on some neutrophil functions. Arch Immunol Ther Exp 1998;46:183–92.
12. Costa-Farre C, Prades M, Ribera T, et al. Does intraoperative low partial pressure of oxygen increase the risk of surgical infection following exploratory laparotomy in horses? Vet J 2014;200:175–80.
13. Bratzler DW, Houck PM. Antimicrobial prophylaxis for surgery: an advisory statement from the National Surgical Infection Prevention Project. Am J Surg 2005;189:395–404.
14. Bratzler DW, Houck PM. Antimicrobial prophylaxis for surgery: an advisory statement from the National Surgical Infection Prevention Project. Clin Infect Dis 2004;38:1706–15.
15. Horspool LJ, McKellar QA. Disposition of penicillin G sodium following intravenous and oral administration to Equidae. Br Vet J 1995;151:401–12.
16. Love DN, Rose RJ, Martin CA, et al. Serum concentrations of penicillin in the horse after administration of a variety of penicillin preparations. Equine Vet J 1983;15:43–8.
17. Magdesian KG, Hogan P, Cohen ND, et al. Pharmacokinetics of a high dose of gentamicin administered intravenously or intramuscularly to horses. J Am Vet Med Assoc 1998;213:1007–11.
18. Fernandez AH, Monge V, Garcinuno MA. Surgical antibiotic prophylaxis: effect in postoperative infections. Eur J Epidemiol 2001;17:369–74.
19. Walter WP, Weber WR, Marti M, et al. The timing of surgical antimicrobial prophylaxis. Ann Surg 2008;247:918–26.
20. Bratzler DW, Houck PM, Richards C, et al. Use of antimicrobial prophylaxis for major surgery: baseline results from the National Surgical Infection Prevention Project. Arch Surg 2005;140:174–82.
21. Durward-Akhurst SA, Mair TS, Boston R, et al. Comparison of two antimicrobial regimes on the prevalence of incisional infections after colic surgery. Vet Rec 2013;172:287–90.
22. Freeman KD, Southwood LL, Lane J, et al. Post-operative infection, pyrexia and perioperative antimicrobial drug use in surgical colic patients. Equine Vet J 2012;44:476–81.
23. Siddiqui AR, Bernstein JM. Chronic wound infection: facts and controversies. Clin Dermatol 2010;28:519–26.

24. United States Department of Agriculture Report: Equine 2005, Part I: Baseline Reference of Equine Health and Management, 2005. Available at: http://www.aphis.usda.gov/animal_health/nahms/equine/downloads/equine05/Equine05_dr_PartI.pdf. Accessed May, 2017.

25. Hughes LA, Pinchbeck G, Gallaby R, et al. Antimicrobial prescribing practice in UK equine veterinary practice. Equine Vet J 2013;45:141–7.

26. Ross SE, Duz M, Rendle DI. Antimicrobial selection and dosing in the treatment of wounds in the United Kingdom. Equine Vet J 2015;48:676–80.

27. Freeman K, Woods E, Welsby S, et al. Biofilm evidence and the microbial diversity of horse wounds. Can J Microbiol 2009;55:197–202.

28. Westgate SJ, Percival SL, Knottenbelt DC, et al. Microbiology of equine wounds and evidence of bacterial biofilms. Vet Microbiol 2011;150:152–9.

29. Van Hecke LL, Hermans K, Haspeslagh M, et al. A quantitative swab is a good non-invasive alternative to quantitative biopsy for quantifying bacterial load in wounds healing by second intention in horses. Vet J 2017;225:63–8.

30. Fernandes A, Dias M. The microbiological profile of infected prosthetic implants with emphasis on which organism form biofilms. J Clin Diagn Res 2013;7:219–23.

31. Leaper D, Assadian O, Edmiston CE. Approach to chronic wound infections. Br J Dermatol 2010;173:351–8.

32. Weese JS, Baptiste KE, Baverud V, et al. Guidelines for antimicrobial use in horses. Oxford (England): Blackwell Publishing; 2008. p. 161–9.

33. Wilson WD. Rational selection of antimicrobials for use in horses. Proc Am Assoc Equine Pract Ann Conv 2001;47:75–93.

34. Rubio-Martinez LM, Elmasi CR, Black B, et al. Clinical use of antimicrobial regional limb perfusion in horses: 174 cases (1999-2009). J Am Vet Med Assoc 2012;241:1650–8.

35. Schneider RK, Bramlage LR, Moore RM, et al. A retrospective study of 192 horses affected with septic arthritis/tenosynovitis. Equine Vet J 1992;24:436–42.

36. Orsini JA. Management of severely infected wounds. In: Stashak TS, Theoret C, editors. Equine wound management. 2nd edition. Ames (IA): Wiley-Blackwell; 2008. p. 543–67.

37. Dart JA, Sole-Guitart A, Stashak TS, et al. Management practices that influence wound infection and healing. In: Theoret C, Schumacher J, editors. Equine wound management. 3rd edition. Ames (IA): John Wiley & Sons, Inc; 2017. p. 47–74.

38. Orsini JA, Elce YA, Kraus B. Management of severely infected wounds. In: Theoret C, Schumacher J, editors. Equine wound management. 3rd edition. Ames (IA): John Wiley & Sons, Inc; 2017. p. 449–75.

39. Levine DG, Epstein KL, Ahern BJ, et al. Efficacy of three tourniquet types for intravenous antimicrobial regional limb perfusion in standing horses. Vet Surg 2010; 39:1021–4.

40. Alkabes SB, Adams SB, Moore GE, et al. Comparison of two tourniquets and determination of amikacin sulfate concentrations after metacarpophalangeal joint lavage performed simultaneously with intravenous regional limb perfusion in horses. AM J Vet Res 2011;72:613–9.

41. Levine DG, Epstein KL, Neelis DA, et al. Effect of topical application of 1% diclofenac sodium liposomal cream on inflammation in healthy horses undergoing intravenous regional limb perfusion with amikacin sulfate. Am J Vet Res 2009; 70:1323–5.

42. Parra-Sanchez A, Lugo J, Boothe DM, et al. Pharmacokinetics and pharmacodynamics of enrofloxacin and low dose amikacin administered via regional limb perfusion in standing horses. Am J Vet Res 2006;67:1687–95.

43. Lallemand E, Trencart P, Tahier C, et al. Pharmacokinetics, pharmacodynamics and local tolerance at injection site of marbofloxacin administered by regional limb perfusion in standing horses. Vet Surg 2013;42:649–57.

44. Hyde RM, Lynch TM, Clark CK, et al. The influence of perfusate volume on antimicrobial concentrations in synovial fluid following intravenous regional limb perfusion in the standing horse. Can Vet J 2013;54:363–7.

45. Kelmer G, Tatz A, Kdoshimi E, et al. Evaluation of the pharmacokinetics of imipenem following regional limb perfusion using the saphenous and cephalic veins in standing horses. Res Vet Sci 2017;114:64–8.

46. Stashak TS, Theoret C. Integumentary system. In: Orsini JA, Divers TJ, editors. Equine emergencies: treatment and procedures. 3rd edition. St Louis (MO): Elsevier; 2008. p. 189–236.

47. Edwards R, Harding KG. Bacteria and wound healing. Curr Opin Infect Dis 2004; 17:91–6.

48. Menke NB, Ward KR, Witten TM. Impaired wound healing. Clin Dermatol 2007;25: 19–25.

49. Marshal JF, Blikslager AT. The effect of non-steroidal anti-inflammatory drugs on the equine intestine. Equine Vet J Suppl 2011;39:140–4.

50. Hamm D, Turchi P, Johnson JC, et al. Determination of an effective dose of eltenac and its comparison with that of flunixin meglumine in horses after experimentally induced carpitis. Am J Vet Res 1997;58:298–302.

51. Johnson CB, Taylor PM, Young SS. Postoperative analgesia using phenylbutazone, flunixin or carprofen in horses. Vet Rec 1993;133:336–8.

52. Kallings P, Johnston C, Drevemo S. Effects of flunixin on movement and performance of standardbred trotters on the track. Equine Vet J 1999;(Suppl 30):270–3.

53. Moses VS, Bertone AL. Nonsteroidal anti-inflammatory drugs. Vet Clin N Am-Equine 2002;18:21–7.

54. Dong YL, Fleming RYD, Yan TZ, et al. Effect of ibuprofen on the inflammatory response to surgical wounds. J Trauma 1993;35:340–3.

55. Dvivedi S, Tiwari SM, Sharma A. Effect of ibuprofen and diclofenac sodium on experimental wound healing. Indian J Exp Biol 1997;35:1243–5.

56. Krischak GD, Augat P, Claes L, et al. The effects of non-steroidal anti-inflammatory drug application on incisional wound healing in rats. J Wound Care 2007;16: 76–8.

57. Jones MK, Wang H, Peskar BM, et al. Inhibition of angiogenesis by nonsteroidal anti-inflammatory drugs: insight into mechanisms and implications for cancer growth and ulcer healing. Nat Med 1999;5:1418–23.

58. Gorman HA, Wolf WA, Frost WW, et al. The effects of oxyphenylbutazone on surgical wounds of the horse. J Am Vet Med Assoc 1968;152:487–91.

59. Robinson NE. Table of common drugs and appropriate dosages. In: Sprayberry KA, Robinson NE, editors. Current therapy in equine medicine. 7th edition. St. Louis (MO): Elsevier; 2015. p. 933–53.

60. Brayton CF. Dimethylsulfoxide (DMSO): a review. Cornell Vet 1986;76:61–90.

61. Welch RD, DeBowes RM, Liepold HW. Evaluation of the effects of intra-articular injection of dimethylsulfoxide on normal equine articular tissues. Am J Vet Res 1989;50:1180–2.

62. Alsup EM, DeBowes RM. Dimethylsulfoxide. J Am Vet Med Assoc 1984;9:1011–4.

63. Welch RD, Watkins JP, DeBowes RM, et al. Effects of intra-articular administration of dimethylsulfoxide on chemically induced synovitis in immature horses. Am J Vet Res 1991;52:934–9.
64. Cimetti LJ, Merriam JG, D'Oench SN. How to perform intravenous regional limb perfusion using amikacin and DMSO. Amer Assoc Equine Pract Ann Conv 2004;50:219–23.

Regenerative Medicine Therapies for Equine Wound Management

Linda A. Dahlgren, DVM, PhD

KEYWORDS

- Regenerative medicine • Wound healing • Low-level laser therapy • Hyaluronic acid
- Scaffold • Amniotic membrane • Stem cell • Platelet-rich plasma

KEY POINTS

- Regenerative medicine provides promising new tools for equine wound management.
- Regenerative therapies can function as scaffolds, cells, and bioactive factors or a combination of these building blocks of tissue regeneration.
- Regenerative therapies such as acellular extracellular matrix scaffolds, cross-linked hyaluronic acid, platelet-rich plasma, low-level laser therapy, and allogeneic amniotic membrane can be readily incorporated into routine equine wound management.
- Regulatory and safety concerns should be considered in selecting a therapy.
- Regenerative medicine therapies should be used in conjunction with, not in the place of, the application of good wound healing practices and serial reassessment of the wound.

INTRODUCTION

Wound management in horses can strike fear in some and passion in others. Wounds are common injuries in horses of all descriptions and require exceptional knowledge and care to achieve a successful outcome. Not all decisions are difficult, but they do require serial attention to detail from the time of initial presentation through what can be a long and intricate series of decisions based on wound progression and desired cosmetic outcome. New treatments to overcome the critical challenges with equine wounds are always desired: managing dehisced and/or nonhealing wounds, managing exuberant granulation tissue, and ultimately achieving functional tissue coverage. A good cosmetic outcome is a bonus. Regenerative medicine represents a broad set of tools with great promise to manipulate the deficiencies recognized in equine wound healing and improve the outcome.[1,2]

This chapter is dedicated to Dr Larry C. Booth, Jr, DVM, MS, Diplomate ACVS. Larry meticulously taught me about equine wound management. His passion for wound healing was infectious, and I am proud to share his teachings with my patients, their owners, and my students. Larry will be missed, but his legacy lives on.
Department of Large Animal Clinical Sciences, Virginia-Maryland College of Veterinary Medicine, Virginia Tech, Blacksburg, 205 Duck Pond Drive, VA 24061-0442, USA
E-mail address: lad11@vt.edu

REGENERATIVE MEDICINE

Regenerative medicine, in its most general terms, refers to the creation of tissues to replace or restore native tissues that are absent, lost, or damaged due to congenital defect, aging, disease, or injury. This definition covers a vast range of therapies. One of the most dramatic and publicized examples of regenerative therapies is the successful engineering of a fully functional urinary bladder from autologous urothelial and smooth muscle cells and a bladder-shaped biodegradable polymer[3] for human patients. More simple examples of regenerative medicine are used in human and veterinary medicine on a daily basis (eg, platelet-rich plasma [PRP] and autologous conditioned serum). The field of regenerative therapies is expanding at such a rapid pace that it is difficult to keep up with new scientific findings and indeed the applications of various therapies has even outpaced the rate at which evidence-based medicine can provide data to support clinical applications. Outpacing the ability to produce rigorous evidence of efficacy is certainly true for regenerative therapies used for equine wound management.

REGENERATIVE MEDICINE IN WOUND HEALING

Regenerative therapies can be broadly divided into 3 categories based on proposed mechanism of action in wound healing: (1) scaffold-based therapies; (2) cell-based therapies; and (3) those that provide bioactive factors that direct the healing process (**Box 1**). Wound healing is a complex physiologic process requiring orchestration of contributions from the extracellular matrix, the cells that produce extracellular matrix (granulation tissue and epithelium), and the cells responsible for producing the bioactive factors that function to recruit other endogenous cells, and to dictate the proteins they in turn produce. As a result of the complexity of the process, it is inherent that some therapies contribute in more than one way to the healing process.

Scaffolds

An extracellular matrix scaffold is essential for structural support to a wound and to provide a physical framework suitable for cell adhesion and migration into the defect

---

Box 1
Examples of regenerative medicine therapies for wound healing based on mechanism of action

Scaffolds
  ACell Vet[a]
  Platelet-rich plasma (PRP)
  Hyaluronic acid (HA)
  Amniotic membrane

Cells
  Mesenchymal stem cells
  Peripheral blood-derived stem cells
  Induced pluripotent stem cells

Bioactive Factors
  ACell Vet[a]
  PRP
  HA
  Amniotic membrane
  Mesenchymal stem cells

  [a] ACell, Inc, Columbia, MD.

for healing to progress. In its purest form during first intention healing, this scaffold is limited to a small blood clot. However, in second intention wound healing, where a substantial deficit or void can be present early in wound healing, structural support is especially important. This void must first be filled with a provisional scaffold before wound healing can progress through contraction and epithelialization. Because of the traumatic nature of many equine wounds, and associated tissue loss, management of wounds by second intention healing is common. Careful management of native scaffold, primarily granulation tissue, throughout the healing process can be advantageous to achieve success. Regenerative medicine products capable of functioning as a temporary, early scaffold and those that stimulate the formation of granulation tissue can be useful tools in wound management.

Cell-Based Therapies

Cells are the work horses of the wound healing process. Fibroblasts excrete extracellular matrix—collagen and glycosaminoglycans—and myofibroblasts result in wound contracture. White blood cells contribute to wound debridement, cell recruitment, and stimulation of matrix production. Regenerative medicine approaches to wound healing include the use of mesenchymal stem cells (MSC) in various forms with the aim of providing trophic mediators capable of stimulating and orchestrating an improved healing response. MSC delivered to the site of injury may also contribute to healing through differentiation into mature cells types, such as fibroblasts, that contribute directly to healing.

Bioactive Factors

The term "bioactive factors" refers to a diverse assembly of growth factors and cytokines that are essential for healing progression at the site of injury. Immediately after injury, chemokines signal white blood cells, MSC, and fibroblasts and recruit them to the wound. Growth factors and cytokines direct the healing response as it progresses, recruiting additional cells and stimulating those already present to an overall anabolic state. Optimal healing relies on chemical signaling to first moderate and then curtail inflammation later in the healing process. Prolonged inflammation results in the formation of exuberant granulation tissue and undesirable scar tissue formation. As healing progresses, growth factors play a key role in stimulating the proliferation and migration of epithelial cells critical for wound closure.

REGENERATIVE MEDICINE THERAPIES FOR USE IN EQUINE PRACTICE

Many exciting therapies are under investigation for wound healing applications in human and veterinary medicine. There is substantial promise that many of these products will ultimately become available and be economically feasible for clinical application in horses. At the present time, there are limited practical options. The remainder of this article focuses on the most relevant and currently available treatment options that can broadly be considered "regenerative" in nature. This implies products whose mechanism of action relies on a specific host response to achieve a successful outcome that is superior to that which would be achieved through standard wound management alone, whether that be increased rate of healing or improved quality of healing.

Acellular Extracellular Matrix Products

Acellular extracellular matrix bioscaffolds were developed more than 30 years ago and have been used for a wide range of tissue repair applications in human and veterinary medicine.[4] Following removal of the immunogenic cellular component, these xenoge-neic products (primary of porcine origin) contain both structural and functional mole-cules important in tissue repair, including collagen, glycosaminoglycans, growth factors, chemokines, and cytokines. Constructive remodeling begins within 2 days of implantation and continues for months characterized by a robust macrophage response, which shifts from a primarily inflammatory (M1) macrophage phenotype in the first few days to a predominantly antiinflammatory or prohealing (M2) macrophage response after 1 to 2 weeks.[4] Peptides released during remodeling can have bioactive effects, including angiogenesis, and promotion of cell migration, adhesion, and differ-entiation, as well as antimicrobial effects.[4] The beneficial effects of acellular bio-scaffolds on tissue regeneration are well-documented and are clearly applicable to equine wound healing. A major advantage of such products is that the full biochemical complexity of the native proteins is retained following the decellularization process, providing a physiologically relevant combination of proteins. ACell Vet (ACell, Inc, Columbia, MD) is an off-the-shelf product derived from porcine bladder basement membrane and is available in a lyophilized (freeze dried) sheet that lends itself well to wound applications. The lyophilized sheet is easy to apply and can be maintained under a bandage for several days.

Hyaluronic Acid

Hyaluronic acid (HA) is a nonsulfated glycosaminoglycan present throughout the body tissues and is important in the structure and organization of extracellular matrix.[5] HA also plays a role in cell proliferation, differentiation, adhesion, and migration and directly mediates effects important in wound healing, such as production of proinflam-matory cytokines, cell proliferation, and the organization of the extracellular matrix of granulation tissue.[6,7] Native HA is degraded rapidly and has poor structural properties. However, when chemically modified to form a stronger product that is more resistant to degradation, the resulting cross-linked HA-based biomaterials provide an excellent tool for wound healing. Equine wounds treated with a cross-linked HA film preparation (equitrX, SentrX Animal Health, Salt Lake City, UT) (**Figs. 1** and **2**) healed faster and with a higher quality, less fragile epithelium than control wounds.[6,8] Repeated applica-tion of the gel formulation of this product (equitrX, SentrX Animal Health, Salt Lake City, UT) was proposed as a treatment option to help stimulate the formation of healthy granulation tissue in the early healing of wounds with large defects.[6] The gel (equitrX, SentrX Animal Health, Salt Lake City, UT) is available in a convenient spray bottle for easy application (see **Figs. 1** and **2**).

Low-Level Laser Therapy

Low-level laser therapy (LLLT) is a form of photobiomodulation, in other words, the application of light to a tissue to promote healing, reduce inflammation, and relieve pain.[9] The effects are not caused by the generation of heat, but by the absorption of energy in the form of light, which then causes a chemical change in the cells (likely within the mitochondria) within the treated tissue. LLLT stimulates myofibroblast gen-eration, collagen deposition, and keratinocyte proliferation and reduces oxidative stress and inflammation. Although numerous, studies on wound healing in general are difficult to summarize due to a wide range of equipment and protocols used. In general, LLLT is a highly effective treatment for acute and chronic wounds of various pathologies and across a variety of species. Care should be taken to observe appro-priate laser safety and to follow guidelines provided with the individual laser to be used. Using an appropriate dose is important, because under- or overdosing can result in less than optimal results. The 3 commonly used dose parameters are time,

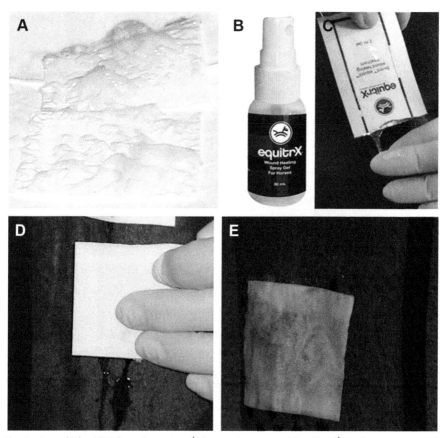

Fig. 1. Cross-linked HA-based products[b] for equine wound healing ([b]equitrX, SentrX Animal Health, Salt Lake City, UT). (*A*) Cross-linked HA film[b] preparation that has been moistened with saline for the purpose of showing the HA film detaching from the nonstick pad to which it was cast during manufacturing. In practice, films are applied dry and become moistened naturally by wound exudate. (*B, C*) Cross-linked HA gel[b] preparation in a convenient spray bottle and the foil pouch used for the experimental study described.[6] (*D, E*) Cross-linked HA film[b] preparation applied to an experimental wound before bandage application and 3 days later at bandage removal. (1B and 1C *courtesy of* SentrX Animal Care, Inc, Salt Lake City, UT; with permission.)

energy, and energy density, but there is no agreed-on method for calculating dose. It is best to refer to the protocols for specific applications provided by the manufacturer with an individual unit because the physics will vary between manufacturers and class of laser. Class 3B lasers are a good choice for veterinary medicine and are available in portable, battery-operated units that are easy to use in the field (**Fig. 3**). For equine wound healing, a large light-emitting diode (LED) cluster probe with multiple diodes at different wavelengths is ideal because a large surface area can be covered at one time (see **Fig. 3**). The LED cluster probe can be used around the margins of the wound to decrease swelling and edema as well as directly over the wound itself to promote tissue healing (see **Fig. 3**). A single control unit can be used to power a variety of probes, including the LED cluster probe, higher-energy infrared single laser probes,

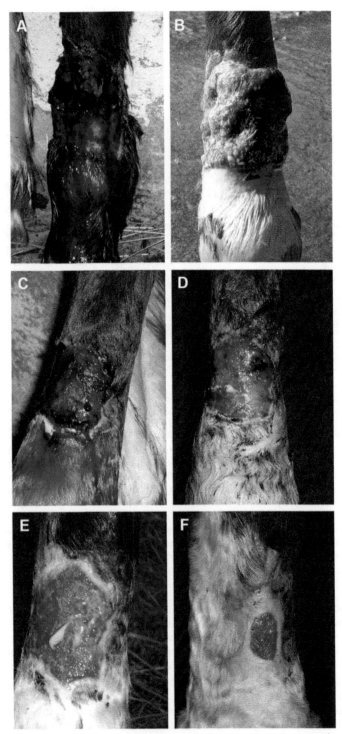

Fig. 2. Example of a clinical wound treated with the cross-linked HA film[b] preparation ([b]equitrX, SentrX Animal Health, Salt Lake City, UT). (*A*) Original wound over the dorsal

and infrared laser cluster probes. The higher-power infrared single laser and laser cluster probes should not be used on open wounds because the intensely focused energy they deliver will damage the healing tissue. Typical treatment times are 30 to 60 seconds per application site and are repeated 2 to 3 times per week for 2 to 3 weeks to achieve the desired effect.

Platelet-Rich Plasma

The term "platelet-rich plasma" is used loosely to refer to a host of blood products generally made from the same horse that has the wound to be treated (autologous). The commonality of these products is that they are made from anticoagulant-treated blood (plasma) in which the red blood cells have largely been removed and the platelets are then concentrated to a variable extent in the plasma fraction. The white blood cell concentration in these products varies widely based on the method used to produce the PRP and can range from leukocyte-poor or leukocyte-depleted to leukocyte-rich. The principals of PRP nomenclature and production are reviewed elsewhere.[10,11] The number of platelets required and whether the absence or presence of white blood cells is desirable for a particular clinical application is up for debate.[11,12]

The principals of PRP application to wound healing include the presence of a biological scaffold in the form of fibrin[10] from the plasma fraction and delivery of a physiologic mixture of growth factors and cytokines contained within the platelets (and white blood cells). The alpha granules of platelets contain high concentrations of growth factors important in tissue repair: platelet-derived growth factor, transforming growth factor beta 1 (TGF-β1), epidermal growth factor, and vascular endothelial growth factor.[13] Once stimulated, platelets degranulate, releasing these growth factors into the surrounding pericellular or vascular environment. The amount of growth factor released from PRP is correlated to the number of platelets and how completely the degranulation occurs.[14,15]

Both commercial and manual methods of making PRP are currently available, making it an accessible regenerative therapy for general equine practice. The cost of making PRP depends on the system used, but is fairly inexpensive, ranging from the cost of the disposables and anticoagulant for manual methods to several hundred dollars for the disposables used in commercial systems. Manual methods require a simple, standard centrifuge capable of holding standard blood tubes, whereas many commercial systems require a proprietary centrifuge and/or rotor. When applied topically to an open wound, the method of making PRP may be more forgiving than PRP preparation for intratendinous and intraarticular injection. An equine wound is generally contaminated, whereas the utmost care in sterile technique and product is required for orthopedic applications. Although the presence of leukocytes may be undesirable in some orthopedic applications, wound healing applications require a completely different set

---

metatarsus, including laceration of the digital extensor tendon. (*B*) Wound 8 weeks later showing complete coverage of the wound with exuberant granulation tissue. (*C*) Wound pictured in *B* following sharp excision of the exuberant granulation tissue. Note the healthy granulation bed and small amount of new epithelium at the wound margins. (*D*) Three weeks later exuberant granulation tissue was again trimmed, but healing has not shown substantial progression since the previous evaluation. At this time, a cross-linked HA film[b] was applied and a standard support bandage applied. (*E*) Five days later the wound again had a healthy granulation bed and a new rim of epithelium was visible advancing over the granulation tissue. (*F*) Approximately 3 weeks later most of the wound was covered by healthy epithelium with only a small granulation bed remaining.

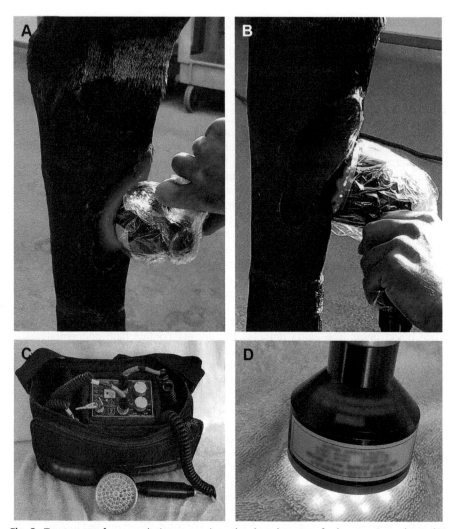

Fig. 3. Treatment of a granulating wound on the dorsal tarsus of a horse using a large (69 diode) light-emitting diode (LED) cluster probe. The probe has been covered with plastic wrap to keep it clean and is being applied to the wound surface (*A*) as well as to the adjacent intact skin (*B*) to reduce soft tissue swelling. Reduced soft tissue swelling reduces pain associated with the wound as well as skin tension, enabling continued reduction in wound size by contraction. A portable control unit (*C*) drives the LED cluster probe consisting of 34 individual 10 mW LEDs at 660 nM and 35 individual 15 mW LEDs at 950 nm (*C, D*).

of considerations. White blood cells in PRP are considered beneficial to wound healing, because they can facilitate wound debridement, produce a physiologic mixture of growth factors and cytokines important in wound healing, and contribute important antibacterial properties.[16,17]

PRP can be applied directly to a wound as a topical "medication" or it can be injected subcutaneously around the wound margins. No tried and true technique for PRP injection is available; however, subcutaneous injection of 2.5 mL along each of the 2-cm long margins of experimental wounds has been described.[18] For topical application, PRP is commonly activated to form a gel before application and held in place by a standard bandage consisting of a nonadherent inner layer and outer supportive layer. Methods of activation include calcium gluconate, thrombin (autologous, bovine, or human), and/or calcium chloride.[19–23] Calcium gluconate or calcium chloride is the recommended method of platelet activation to achieve maximal growth factor release and for biological safety.[24,25] Of these, calcium gluconate may be preferred because it results in efficient platelet degranulation without the formation of the salt precipitates that can form when using calcium chloride.[25]

Clinical reports and experimental studies investigating the use of PRP to improve wound healing in various animal species and people are plentiful; however, studies in the horse are limited and are often only case reports or small case series. No large, controlled clinical trials exist. In a recent meta-analysis evaluating experimentally induced skin wounds in animals, only 2 equine studies met the inclusion criteria.[26] In 2003, PRP gel was reported to accelerate epithelial differentiation and improve collagen organization in experimental full-thickness skin wounds on the metacarpi and metatarsi compared with control wounds treated with either dry or saline-soaked gauze.[21] This study only included a single horse in the study, and as such must be considered with caution when applying the results to the equine population as a whole. Platelet gel applied to experimental wounds on the neck of 6 horses resulted in more rapid epithelialization and increased dermal collagen organization compared with untreated controls.[22] The wounds used in this study consisted of a surgical incision, undermining of the subcutaneous tissue, and primary closure, which may not be a realistic model for most of the wounds for which one might consider PRP application.

PRP gel has been evaluated for full-thickness metacarpal wounds (including excision of the subcutaneous tissue) in horses.[19] Wounds treated with PRP gel developed more exuberant granulation tissue than control wounds and were slower to heal at 1, 2, and 3 weeks after surgery. There were no histologic, biomechanical, or gene expression differences between PRP-treated and control wounds. Concentrations of TGF-β1 were 1.6-fold higher in PRP-treated wounds compared with controls 1 week following treatment. The investigators speculated that the prolonged expression of TGF-β1 may have led to the development of exuberant granulation tissue and that PRP treatment might be better suited to wounds with tissue loss requiring filling with granulation tissue and/or chronic wounds requiring a fresh source of anabolic factors to stimulate the healing process. Other, more recent, studies reporting the use of PRP in horses have used a dermal burn model,[20] gluteal wounds,[27] neck wounds,[28] or reported a single, anecdotal case.[23,29]

Taken together, these studies generally fail to show a beneficial effect of PRP gel on equine wound healing despite a logical theoretic basis for its use. When considering the use of PRP for management of an equine wound, the risk is generally low for topical application of gel, because adverse events have not been reported when autologous PRP was used. Frequency and timing of application and preferred method of preparation are largely unknown, and the potential for the formation of exuberant granulation tissue should be considered based on the nature of the individual wound to be treated.

Amniotic Membrane

Amniotic membrane, the innermost layer of the placenta, is composed of 3 layers: a thin epithelial layer, a thick basement membrane, and avascular mesenchymal tissue.[30,31] Essentially, amnion is a collagen-rich matrix that includes proteoglycans, HA, laminin, growth factors, and heparin sulfate. Whether cells (MSC and epithelial cells) remain present and whether growth factors remain active when applied to a wound depends on the method of preparation and the duration and method of storage. Theoretic benefits of amnion include antiinflammatory, bacteriostatic, reepithelializing, and scar-preventing properties.[32] The structural matrix, preserved regardless of processing and storage, retains potential beneficial properties of tissue scaffolds when used as a biological dressing. The exact mechanisms by which amnion my promote wound healing remain the focus of active investigations.

Amnion has been used for a variety of applications in human and veterinary medicine since the early 1900s, including skin grafts, corneal grafts, surgical dressings, and tissue reconstruction. Reports on the use of amnion on equine wounds are limited, but promising.[33,34] Application of amnion to experimental wounds on the metacarpi and metatarsi of horses resulted in increased percentage of epithelialization and decreased number of days to complete healing compared with control wounds treated with a nonadherent dressing alone.[33] In addition, wounds treated with amnion also had significantly less exuberant granulation tissue compared with controls.[33] In a similar study using amnion as a biological dressing following pinch skin grafting of experimental distal limb wounds, amnion-treated wounds had decreased formation of exuberant granulation tissue and decreased median healing time compared with nonadherent dressing alone.[34] Proteomic analysis of equine amniotic membrane has recently provided initial confirmation of the presence of many of the structural and functional proteins thought to play a role in wound healing.[35] Available evidence suggests that if one has access to equine placentas for the harvest and storage of amnion, allogeneic amnion has low immunogenicity and the potential to enhance wound healing.

Recently, a line of new products derived from equine amnion have become commercially available.[36] These allogeneic products include off-the-shelf, decellularized, lyophilized sheets and pulverized powder for topical and injectable applications. Anecdotal evidence suggests that these products result in rapid formation of granulation tissue and promote wound contraction (**Fig. 4**). Preliminary data support accelerated healing of equine distal limb wounds.[37]

Stem Cells

Stem cell therapies have been at the forefront of regenerative medicine–related news in veterinary medicine since the early 2000s when Dr Herthel first described the use of bone marrow aspirate to treat suspensory desmitis in the horse.[38] Since that time, the use of MSC for the treatment of tendon and ligament injuries has become somewhat commonplace. The idea that stem cells, whether from bone marrow aspirate, fat tissue, peripheral blood, or even induced from fetal skin, are capable of helping achieve faster wound healing and/or better quality scar tissue is appealing.[1,2,39–41] Through direct injection, or use of stem cells in combination with a scaffold and/or growth factor to engineer a replacement skin tissue, stem cell therapy holds good promise.

There is no currently available, successful, off-the-shelf skin replacement for skin graft material. Partial success in human medicine may eventually help deliver such a product to the equine market, but to-date none is available. In vitro work is focused on developing induced pluripotent stem cells that can be differentiated into skin cells.[42] The prospect of using stem cells to deliver secreted factors capable of promoting wound healing in general[43] or through the inhibition of the profibrotic effects of TGF-β1 is also a goal for clinical application.[44]

A single in vivo study has reported the use of allogeneic MSC from equine umbilical cord blood delivered to experimental wounds either in an autologous fibrin gel or injected subcutaneously at the wound margin in 6 horses.[45] Wounds were bandaged

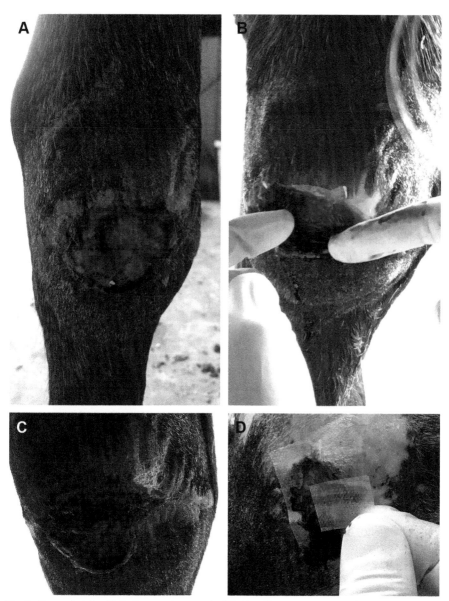

Fig. 4. Example of a clinical wound treated with the allogeneic amnion-derived lyophilized sheet[c] ([c]AniCell Biotech, Chandler, AZ). (*A*) Original wound over the dorsal tarsus before debridement. (*B*) Following debridement the amnion-derived sheet was cut to size and placed over the entire surface of the wound. (*C*) Four days later the bandage was changed and what had been a chronic, static wound showed evidence of new granulation tissue formation, the first step toward reinvigorating the wound healing process. (*D*) An example of a different wound showing better detail of the allogeneic amnion-derived lyophilized sheet[c] used in the wound in *A–C*. (*Courtesy of* Dr Mike Cissell, Prescott, AZ; with permission.)

for 1 week and then left unbandaged to reduce the incidence of exuberant granulation tissue formation that occurred when the wounds were bandaged in pilot studies. Unfortunately, wound healing was confounded by fly irritation and self-mutilation in some horses. MSC injection resulted in significantly increased TGF-β1 and cyclooxygenase-2 (COX-2) gene expression at 1 week as compared with topical MSC-fibrin gel treatment.[45] These changes in gene expression did not persist beyond 1 week. Although considered a hallmark of inflammation, COX-2 is a critical component of early wound healing, and the lack of prolonged TGF-β1 expression could be a marker of uncomplicated rather than dysregulated healing.[45] Histologic (both MSC-treated groups) and histomorphometric (MSC-injected group) analyses showed modest improvements.[45] The routine use of stem cells in any form in equine wound management seems to show promise but is currently an imperfect practice. Cost of MSC treatment is also an important consideration.

Regulatory Considerations

Awareness of regulatory concerns is important when considering regenerative therapies because of their biological origins. The pace of commercial development and clinical use of the various regenerative therapies has, to some extent, moved faster than the regulatory machinery meant to oversee the safety and efficacy of the products. The US Food and Drug Administration (FDA) Center for Veterinary Medicine (CVM) issued Guidance #218 in 2015,[46] which clarifies that cell-based products generally meet the definition of a new animal drug and are therefore subject to the same regulatory requirements as other new animal drugs. This Guidance has provided clarity regarding how the FDA views many of these regenerative medicine products and defines the term "cell-based products" as "those articles containing, consisting of, or derived from cells that are intended for implantation, transplantation, infusion, or transfer into an animal recipient,"[46] and therefore meet the definition of a new animal drug. Based on Guidance #218, xenogeneic and allogeneic, and some autologous products—cells and tissue products (eg, xenogeneic bladder-derived, allogeneic amnion-derived, allogeneic cell-based, and many autologous cell-based regenerative medicine therapies) —require premarket review and approval before marketing. In 2016, the FDA CVM issued a Warning Letter to a company stating that their amnion-derived products were a new animal drug and therefore required approval before marketing.[47] The challenge for the consumer is in knowing what the FDA approval status of an individual product might be, because this information is confidential and, unless it is shared publicly by the company marketing the product, is not available to the public. Autologous products, such as PRP and autologous stem cells are classified as either Type I (more than minimally manipulated, combined with another agent, drug, or device, etc.) or Type II (essentially involves none of the items described as making them Type I). Most regenerative therapies currently on the market require FDA approval based on the definitions put forth in Guidance #218. One important criteria described is whether a product is intended for "homologous use," essentially whether the product is performing the same basic function in the recipient as is in the donor. Based on these definitions, and the complexity of the topic, it is clear that veterinarians and owners need additional information to determine the appropriate use of regenerative medicine therapies in practice. Education and communication from professional associations, industry, and academia are required to improve communication and awareness of these important regulations. At present, one is advised to proceed with caution regarding the selection of any regenerative medicine therapies for clinical use. There are currently no FDA-approved regenerative medicine cell-based products; therefore, the onus is on

---

Box 2
Ways to incorporate regenerative medicine therapies into your practice

1. Off-the-shelf acellular extracellular matrix products such as ACell Vet[a] or cross-linked HA gel[b]

2. Off-the-shelf amniotic membrane products such as AniCell[c]

3. Identify a PRP system that uses an existing centrifuge in your practice
   a. Centrifuge that holds standard blood tubes
   b. Centrifuge for processing IRAP serum[d]

4. Invest in a good-quality Class 3B laser system with a large LED cluster probe designed for wound healing applications

[a] ACell, Inc, Columbia, MD.
[b] equitrX, SentrX Animal Health, Salt Lake City, UT.
[c] AniCell Biotech, Chandler, AZ.
[d] ORTHOGEN Veterinary GmbH, Düsseldorf, Germany.

---

the veterinarian to know the donor selection and manufacturing practices used to produce a product and to perform due diligence with respect to FDA approval status and, more importantly, any safety data associated with an individual product. Whether a product is efficacious or not is an entirely separate, and equally gray, subject. It is of the utmost importance that a product be safe, but it is also imperative that owners receive an unbiased presentation of any available evidence-based information regarding product efficacy before deciding how to spend their money.

SUMMARY

When faced with a wounded horse, formulation of an immediate treatment plan is critical, but the long-term goals and related plan to achieve those goals must also be taken under consideration when making critical decisions. Critical factors include wound location and severity, the intended use of the horse, owner finances, and the temperament of the horse. There is no substitute for careful application of the basic, conventional principles of wound healing and management. The currently available regenerative therapies have the potential to be excellent complementary tools that may be useful at specific stages of wound healing (**Box 2**).

Serial reassessment of a healing wound is critical to achieve a successful outcome. There is no substitute for understanding what to expect from a particular type of wound. When a wound deviates from "normal" progression, which they often do, the wound should be reassessed to identify a reason for the change and hopefully modify the treatment plan to get healing back on track. Each regenerative therapy, just like conventional therapies, is likely to have an ideal application or timing of application for the best outcome. A successful outcome is achievable with many wounds using common sense and conventional approaches. Regenerative therapies definitely have a place in the treatment of equine wounds. Controlled clinical trials and well-documented case series are required to provide much stronger evidence-based literature to better support the development and integration of regenerative therapies.

REFERENCES

1. Theoret C. Tissue engineering in wound repair: the three "R"s—repair, replace, regenerate. Vet Surg 2009;38(8):905–13.

2. Theoret C. Innovative adjunctive approaches to wound management. In: Theoret C, Schumacher J, editors. Equine wound management. 3rd edition. Ames (IA): Wiley; 2017. p. 508–39.

3. Oberpenning F, Meng J, Yoo JJ, et al. De novo reconstitution of a functional mammalian urinary bladder by tissue engineering. Nat Biotechnol 1999;17(2): 149–55.

4. Swinehart IT, Badylak SF. Extracellular matrix bioscaffolds in tissue remodeling and morphogenesis. Dev Dyn 2016;245(3):351–60.

5. Luo Y, Kirker KR, Prestwich GD. Cross-linked hyaluronic acid hydrogel films: new biomaterials for drug delivery. J Control Release 2000;69(1):169–84.

6. Dahlgren LA, Milton SC, Boswell SG, et al. Evaluation of a hyaluronic acid-based biomaterial to enhance wound healing in the equine distal limb. J Equine Vet Sci 2016;44:90–9.

7. Hussain Z, Thu HE, Katas H, et al. Hyaluronic acid-based biomaterials: a versatile and smart approach to tissue regeneration and treating traumatic, surgical, and chronic wounds. Polym Rev (Phila Pa) 2017;57(4):594–630.

8. Yang G, Prestwich GD, Mann BK. Thiolated carboxymethyl-hyaluronic-acid-based biomaterials enhance wound healing in rats, dogs, and horses. ISRN Vet Sci 2012;2011:851593.

9. Farivar S, Malekshahabi T, Shiari R. Biological effects of low level laser therapy. J Lasers Med Sci 2014;5(2):58–62.

10. David MDE, Tomasz B, Ryo J, et al. Do the fibrin architecture and leukocyte content influence the growth factor release of platelet concentrates? an evidence-based answer comparing a pure platelet-rich plasma (P-PRP) gel and a leukocyte- and platelet-rich fibrin (L-PRF). Curr Pharm Biotechnol 2012; 13(7):1145–52.

11. McLellan J, Plevin S. Does it matter which platelet-rich plasma we use? Equine Vet Educ 2011;23(2):101–4.

12. Boswell SG, Cole BJ, Sundman EA, et al. Platelet-rich plasma: a milieu of bioactive factors. Arthroscopy 2012;28(3):429–39.

13. Anitua E, Prado R, Orive G. PRP therapies-is it time for potency assays? Letter to the Editor. Am J Sports Med 2016;44(11):NP63–4.

14. Sutter WW, Kaneps AJ, Bertone AL. Comparison of hematologic values and transforming growth factor-beta and insulin-like growth factor concentrations in platelet concentrates obtained by use of buffy coat and apheresis methods from equine blood. Am J Vet Res 2004;65(7):924–30.

15. McCarrel T, Fortier L. Temporal growth factor release from platelet-rich plasma, trehalose lyophilized platelets, and bone marrow aspirate and their effect on tendon and ligament gene expression. J Orthop Res 2009;27(8):1033–42.

16. Bielecki TM, Gazdzik TS, Arendt J, et al. Antibacterial effect of autologous platelet gel enriched with growth factors and other active substances: an in vitro study. J Bone Joint Surg Br 2007;89(3):417–20.

17. Cieslik-Bielecka A, Gazdzik TS, Bielecki TM, et al. Why the platelet-rich gel has antimicrobial activity? Oral Surg Oral Med Oral Pathol Oral Radiol Endod 2007; 103(3):303–5 [author reply: 305–6].

18. Pereira RCdF, De La Côrte FD, Brass KE, et al. Evaluation of three methods of platelet-rich plasma for treatment of equine distal limb skin wounds. J Equine Vet Sci 2017.

19. Monteiro SO, Lepage OM, Theoret CL. Effects of platelet-rich plasma on the repair of wounds on the distal aspect of the forelimb in horses. Am J Vet Res 2009;70(2):277–82.

20. Maciel FB, DeRossi R, Módolo TJC, et al. Scanning electron microscopy and microbiological evaluation of equine burn wound repair after platelet-rich plasma gel treatment. Burns 2012;38(7):1058–65.
21. Carter CA, Jolly DG, Worden CE, et al. Platelet-rich plasma gel promotes differentiation and regeneration during equine wound healing. Exp Mol Pathol 2003; 74(3):244–55.
22. DeRossi R, Coelho ACAdO, Mello GSd, et al. Effects of platelet-rich plasma gel on skin healing in surgical wound in horses. Acta Cir Bras 2009;24:276–81.
23. López C, Carmona JU. Platelet-rich plasma as an adjunctive therapy for the management of a severe chronic distal limb wound in a foal. J Equine Vet Sci 2014; 34(9):1128–33.
24. Textor JA, Tablin F. Activation of equine platelet-rich plasma: comparison of methods and characterization of equine autologous thrombin. Vet Surg 2012; 41(7):784–94.
25. Giraldo CE, Álvarez ME, Carmona JU. Influence of calcium salts and bovine thrombin on growth factor release from equine platelet-rich gel supernatants. Vet Comp Orthop Traumatol 2017;30(01):1–7.
26. Tambella AM, Attili AR, Dupré G, et al. Platelet-rich plasma to treat experimentally-induced skin wounds in animals: a systematic review and meta-analysis. PLoS One 2018;13(1):e0191093.
27. de Souza MV, Silva MB, Pinto JdO, et al. Immunohistochemical expression of collagens in the skin of horses treated with leukocyte-poor platelet-rich plasma. Biomed Res Int 2015;2015:893485.
28. Bonfá AF, Nomura RHC, Prado AMBd, et al. Efeito do gel de plasma rico em plaquetas na cicatrização de enxertos cutâneos em equinos. Ciência Animal Brasileira 2017;18.
29. Iacopetti I, Perazzi A, Ferrari V, et al. Application of platelet-rich gel to enhance wound healing in the horse: a case report. J Equine Vet Sci 2012;32(3):123–8.
30. Mamede AC, Carvalho MJ, Abrantes AM, et al. Amniotic membrane: from structure and functions to clinical applications. Cell Tissue Res 2012;349(2):447–58.
31. Sadler TW. Langman's medical embryology. 13th edition. Baltimore (MD): Lippincott Williams & Wilkins, a Wolters Kluwer business; 2015.
32. Litwiniuk M, Grzela T. Amniotic membrane: new concepts for an old dressing. Wound Repair Regen 2014;22(4):451–6.
33. Bigbie RB, Schumacher J, Swaim SF, et al. Effects of amnion and live yeast cell derivative on second-intention healing in horses. Am J Vet Res 1991;52(8): 1376–82.
34. Goodrich LR, Moll HD, Crisman MV, et al. Comparison of equine amnion and a nonadherent wound dressing material for bandaging pinch-grafted wounds in ponies. Am J Vet Res 2000;61(3):326–9.
35. Galera PD, Ribeiro CR, Sapp HL, et al. Proteomic analysis of equine amniotic membrane: characterization of proteins. Vet Ophthalmol 2015;18(3):198–209.
36. AniCell. Available at: http://anicellbiotech.com/veterinarians/products/equuscell/. Accessed June 9, 2018.
37. Fowler AW, Gilbertie JM, Prange T, et al. Commercially available acellular equine amniotic allografts accelerate healing of experimentally induced full-thickness distal limb wounds in horses compared to silicone dressings or nonadherent dressings. Vet Surg 2017;46:E21.
38. Herthel DJ. Enhanced suspensory ligament healing in 100 horses by stem cells and other bone marrow components. Paper presented at Proc Ann Conv Am Assoc Equine Pract. San Diego, CA, November 25 – 28, 2001.

39. Balaji S, Keswani SG, Crombleholme TM. The role of mesenchymal stem cells in the regenerative wound healing phenotype. Adv Wound Care (New Rochelle) 2012;1(4):159–65.
40. Lee DE, Ayoub N, Agrawal DK. Mesenchymal stem cells and cutaneous wound healing: novel methods to increase cell delivery and therapeutic efficacy. Stem Cell Res Ther 2016;7:37.
41. Borena BM, Martens A, Broeckx SY, et al. Regenerative skin wound healing in mammals: state-of-the-art on growth factor and stem cell based treatments. Cell Physiol Biochem 2015;36(1):1–23.
42. Aguiar C, Therrien J, Lemire P, et al. Differentiation of equine induced pluripotent stem cells into a keratinocyte lineage. Equine Vet J 2016;48(3):338–45.
43. Bussche L, Harman RM, Syracuse BA, et al. Microencapsulated equine mesenchymal stromal cells promote cutaneous wound healing in vitro. Stem Cell Res Ther 2015;6:66.
44. Harman RM, Bihun IV, Van de Walle GR. Secreted factors from equine mesenchymal stromal cells diminish the effects of TGF-beta1 on equine dermal fibroblasts and alter the phenotype of dermal fibroblasts isolated from cutaneous fibroproliferative wounds. Wound Repair Regen 2017;25(2):234–47.
45. Textor JA, Clark KC, Walker NJ, et al. Allogeneic stem cells alter gene expression and improve healing of distal limb wounds in horses. Stem Cells Transl Med 2018; 7(1):98–108.
46. U.S. Department of Health and Human Services FaDA, Center for Veterinary Medicine. #218 Guidance for Industry; Cell-Based Products for Animal Use. 2015. Available at: https://www.fda.gov/downloads/AnimalVeterinary/Guidance ComplianceEnforcement/GuidanceforIndustry/UCM405679.pdf. Accessed June 9, 2018.
47. VetraGenics 8/9/16. Available at: https://www.fda.gov/ICECI/Enforcement Actions/WarningLetters/2016/ucm518593.htm. Accessed June 9, 2018.

Moving?

Make sure your subscription moves with you!

To notify us of your new address, find your **Clinics Account Number** (located on your mailing label above your name), and contact customer service at:

Email: journalscustomerservice-usa@elsevier.com

800-654-2452 (subscribers in the U.S. & Canada)
314-447-8871 (subscribers outside of the U.S. & Canada)

Fax number: 314-447-8029

Elsevier Health Sciences Division
Subscription Customer Service
3251 Riverport Lane
Maryland Heights, MO 63043

*To ensure uninterrupted delivery of your subscription, please notify us at least 4 weeks in advance of move.

Printed and bound by CPI Group (UK) Ltd, Croydon, CR0 4YY

12/10/2024

01773487-0001